FOREVER YOUNG

FOREVER YOUNG

Science and the Search for Immortality

Jim Schnabel

BLOOMSBURY

First published in Great Britain in 1998

Bloomsbury Publishing Plc, 38 Soho Square, London W1V 5DF

Copyright © 1998 by Jim Schnabel

The moral right of the author has been asserted

A CIP catalogue record for this book is available from the British Library

ISBN 0 7475 3704 6

10 9 8 7 6 5 4 3 2 1

Typeset by Palimpsest Book Production Limited,
Polmont, Stirlingshire
Printed in Great Britain by
Clays Ltd, St Ives plc

I don't want to achieve immortality through my works. I want to achieve immortality by not dying.

– Woody Allen

CONTENTS

Thanatopolis   1

Phase One: Forever Old   7

1 Mildred   9
2 Brain 204   14
3 Inflammation   22
4 Voices in the Wilderness   35
5 The Harvard Baptist   45
6 Mac Attack   60
7 The Finish Line   72
8 The Wall   82

Phase Two: Spare Parts   91

9 The Ordeal of Near-Death   93
10 The Secret Handshake   105
11 The Ligand   114
12 The Blocker   123
13 The Grail   130
14 Twelve Monkeys   142
15 We Can All Go Home Now   157
16 The Selfish Self   161

Phase Three: Forever Young   167

17 The Grey Gene   169
18 The Race   174
19 The Markers   182
20 The Gene Cleaner   194
Acknowledgements   210
Source Notes   211
Bibliography   215
Index   226

Thanatopolis

Approaching Phoenix from the north-west, US Route 60 runs through a blur of sand and rock and brush and scrub. The nature documentaries tell us that such a desert is actually a lively place – oh, full of life – but on this harsh, wind-whipped November day it seems a perfect garden of suffering and death. Its dominant flora are tangles of brittle sticks and briars: burr-laden bursage, salt-loving seepweed and saltbush, thorny catclaw and mesquite and paloverde, toxic creosote-bush, pestilential turpentine-tasting snakeweed, and prickly pear cacti with their green bouquets of pain. About the tallest things around are the occasional gnarled Joshua trees – so named by early settlers for their look of agonized supplication – and the severe, crucifix-like saguaro cacti, both of which must endure up to two centuries of torment in this purgatory, where the daytime temperature in summer regularly exceeds 120 degrees Fahrenheit.

There is no water to be seen; there is only the torturous promise of water. Here lie eroded dry gullies where it flows from brief August storms – and there, great cracked patches of barrenness where it eventually pools and evaporates, rising to heaven, leaving alkali salts that kill even the hardiest forms of left-behind life.

Stark brown mountains, unforested, unleavened by snow, watch impassively over this wasteland. A dark pall of wind-blown dust gathers in the far distance and as a traveller moves towards it down the road at eighty hopeless miles an hour, contemplating the end of youth, he considers the oddly existential phrase he was taught as a Catholic schoolboy: Remember, Man, that you are dust, and to dust you shall return.

Ah, youth! said Conrad, saying it all. Firm limbs and tough bones and clear eyes and high spirits, the mind open to promises, to the orgiastic, Promethean, still-infinite future. I am only thirty-three as I write these words but by God I can see easily enough the lines of weather and time, can feel the slowing, the gradual narrowing of existence. How long will it be till I am hobbled by clotted arteries, humiliated by a burnout of brain matter – Alzheimer's, Parkinson's – or tortured slowly by one of the cancers that hang, black and bloated, from my family tree? How long will it be till I succumb to the inevitable, terminal fate of mortals? Doctor, tell me straight: How long have I got?

I have come here to Arizona to seek an answer to that question, that problem, and already I sense that there is more than one problem to face.

The first problem, an obvious one you could say, is death itself. Death is triumphant, today, over medical technology. It is an implacable beast whose advance doctors and scientists can only delay. I will (touch wood) live much longer than early hominids lived but – as I say, with today's technology – I too am doomed by death, the murderer of every known form of life.

The second problem, perhaps less obvious, is the human acceptance of this situation: this situation of inevitable death. It is an acceptance that comes from religion on one side (God didn't mean for our physical bodies to live for ever) and from Darwinian logic on the other (Evolution didn't mean for our physical bodies to live for ever) and from universal experience in between. Death has always been with us. Death just is.

Death will only begin to go from an is to a was when humans no longer accept it as inevitable. And the current popular obsession with extending life suggests, to me, that this conceptual shift has started: from thinking of death as inevitable to thinking of death as preventable, and of ageing – the ultimate weapon of death – as a disease we might cure. With the right technology.

Scientists, I notice, are busy developing that technology now.

Most of these scientists claim not to be aware of this. They say they are aware only that they are fighting specific diseases and conditions: Alzheimer's, vascular disease, transplant rejection, genetic deficiencies. And when I suggest otherwise to them, they scoff. They do not like to think of themselves as participants in a gigantic, hugely ambitious multi-phase project: the goal of which is immortality. They look at me, when I broach such heretical notions, as if I were one of those flaky people, out in California or wherever – one of those flaky people who want to freeze their heads in liquid nitrogen, to be revived at a later date.

But I am not talking about flakiness. I am not talking (though those Californians may not seem so flaky some day) about freezing brains. I am not talking about any of the worthless 'age-extending' elixirs and potions and creams and salves and surgeries on which humans, intelligent people some of them, waste billions of dollars every year. I am instead talking about hard-nosed, peer-reviewed science, and realistic strategies to slow, to stop – to reverse! let us baby-boomers pray – the deep genetic and biochemical processes that now make us wither and die.

I am talking about a future where we are all biologically twenty-five, and have been for centuries.

For now, alas, the old are old; they can only try to act young. As I speed down the desert highway a baby blue Cadillac, driving even faster, roars around me, its riders two grey-haired grandmothers with smiles on their lips. Perhaps they are on their way back from Vegas. Certainly they are almost home. Housing developments are now rising up from the brown deadness of the desert. We are at the frontier of the Sun Cities.

First comes Sun City Grand, brand new, watered and green, still bordered abruptly by dirt. Next comes the more established Sun City West, and it in turn is followed – as Route 60 slows to golf-cart pace amid traffic lights and strip-malls – by the original Sun City, est. 1960, elev. 1,150, with a pop. that ranges from 75,000 in winter to perhaps 20,000 in the crematory heat of summer.

The Sun Cities, with the purest concentrations of senior citizens on the planet, are another sign of the beginning of the end, or the end of the beginning, of human ageing. Here the grey do not stare from rockers in upstairs rooms, while the dust gathers and the young play frenetically below. Here it is the grey who play. The young are not invited – the young, with all their nervous rushing, their pushy clucking and bustling in grocery store checkout lines and at stoplights. Here in the Sun Cities the lives of citizens are permitted to flow at a wise and judicious

pace. And in so far as possible, these lives are filled with sociable
activity.

The people here join clubs. They have ample time for clubs. There are
clubs for woodworking, stone and gemworking, silversmithing, ceramics
and pottery-making, stained-glassworking, leatherworking, knitting,
weaving, painting, dancing, acting, hymn-singing, harp-playing, church-
supporting, foreign affairs-discussing, domestic affairs-discussing, golf,
bowling, tennis, ping pong, handball, swimming, and fishing, to
name a few. At a visitor's centre I am shown a video for prospective
homebuyers, featuring among other things the Sun City Poms,
grannies in glittery purple one-piece suits and opaque flesh-coloured
tights and spangled red cheerleader pom-poms, and one of them – this
woman must be very close to eighty – one of them is doing backflips
and cartwheels on a stage while the others cheer her on.

Outside I watch senior citizens on the roadway shoulders, stooping
– painfully, one imagines – to remove litter, or to plant flowers
or shrubs. (The streets in this enclave of volunteer socialism are
well-kept, and clean even by American suburban standards.) At
night I see them behind the wheels of Sun City 'Sheriff's Posse' cars,
living out long-held dreams of being policemen. They do not carry
guns, and if they encounter serious trouble they must call the real
police from neighbouring towns. But very seldom is there trouble,
for young people are the ones who commit crimes. And there are
just no young people here. Humans under the age of nineteen are
not allowed to reside within the cities' limits, and each house must
have at least one resident aged fifty-five or older. A few years ago, a
Sun City woman brought her two young grandchildren to live with
her after they were orphaned in a tragic accident. They had nowhere
else to go. Nevertheless the woman's neighbours sued and she was
forced to move away.

But however sunny the Sun Cities, however militantly active their
inhabitants, the signs of the Reaper are everywhere. These are not
real cities. They are an extended thanatopolis. They are liable to
frighten a person still relatively young. Their hospitals have no
obstetrics wards, for there are no births, only deaths. When Sun City
citizens are lifted up to be with their Maker, it is only other elderly
folk who flow in to take their earthly places. The Sun City cemetery
– Sunland Memorial, with flowered plots and crypts – is large and
populous, chthonically festive even on the coldest winter days.

Those still living in this city of death and near-death have an elderly sameness about them, a Borg-like uniformity. Senior citizens' hours are kept with such regularity that many local restaurants are full by five-thirty p.m. and closed by eight. The streets creep with ponderous old-person's cars. The local economy is one of dentures and hearing aids, bifocal lenses, hernia girdles, incontinence pads, leg braces, titanium knee and hip joints, wheelchairs, cataract surgery, chiropractors, golf equipment, condos in giant 'adult community complexes', drugs for arthritis and diabetes and high blood pressure and atherosclerosis and every other corporeal ailment, and funeral planning, and mortuarial services.

Yet in Sun City they seem to age and fade as gracefully as one could hope to do. There is beauty here; there are glades and freshets of youthful memory. I am watching a couple in the massive strip-mall parking lot outside the grocery store, loading bags into their car. She is wearing a pink nylon warmup suit; he is similarly dressed in blue. Their hair is grey and their faces are worn but they are tanned and handsome. Through the years that have been etched upon them one can easily see the young couple, Boy and Girl of the Year in some midwestern small town midsummer, symbols of fertility and vitality amid ears of corn and other fruits of field and stream. He was going off to war, and then would join his father's insurance business. She would pine for him until they wed. Now they put the packages in the car slowly, wordlessly. All those years.

All those years almost slip away at night, at Ritter's Chalet, the German restaurant off Grand Avenue. The gregarious man behind the bar, that young man of forty-five or so named Ari, is playing keyboard and sometimes guitar and sometimes even the trumpet, and bantering with the Sun City customers, making the ladies laugh, and singing in his Sammy Davis voice, 'I've got you . . . under my skin . . .' The old couples get up on to the dance floor and the men, they look stiff, they frown slightly with the effort at remembering all the steps, though they are clearly pleased at being able to do so. The wives are loose, happy, in their element. They are girls. Girls love to dance. They even dance the Macarena, with Ari coming out and showing them where to put their hands. And when he plays 'In the Mood' the place comes alive, the men in their double-knit golf shirts and light grey slacks and white old-man's shoes starting to lose their

stiffness; in fact they steer their better-dressed wives around with
sudden deftness, twirling them and swinging them and then cradling
them from behind, holding them close like in the old days.

Still, these are new days, and over Sun City from dawn to dusk
young lieutenants from Luke Air Force Base cavort and carouse
in their F-16s, learning how to dogfight. Now at noon under
bright sunshine one comes up from the south in a broad westward
arc, another following with his fire-control radar, rocking his ship
insouciantly, while the first turns the corner hard, pulling g-forces no
old man could withstand, and his machine makes a certain dreadful,
tearing noise in the warm desert air.

Meanwhile, almost pathetically far below, a new and white and
perfectly dimpled ball rises up in a neat parabola, seems to hang in
that same desert air, then falls with an unheard thump on the grass
in the middle distance, making a series of small bounces, smaller
each time, never quite reaching the yellow driving-range marker
board that says 100.

The grey-haired man in the green shirt shakes his head and tees
up another ball. The wind today is at his back. He should be driving
the ball farther than 100 yards. Much farther. Why, there was a
time . . .

PHASE ONE
FOREVER OLD

1

Mildred

. . . There was a time, on such a course in Sun City, when Mildred Weller played golf every few days. Indeed she was active by any reasonable standard, geriatric or juvenile. She rode horses. She played the piano, not just casually but well. She attended the symphony and opera and chamber music recitals. She crafted excellent needlepoint embroidery. She read widely; she had degrees in Old English and Education and Business Administration. She played tennis. She rowed. She was a great swimmer. She had always been a great swimmer. At the age of fifty-two, living then in northern Maryland, she had proposed raising money for nearby flood victims by making a marathon swim in a country club pool. Members of the local gentry had promised to donate fifty dollars each, something like that, for every lap she swam. They had assumed she wouldn't complete very many laps. But she swam all day. She raised a pile of money.

Mildred's husband, Max*, was an adventurous Byelorussian-Jewish émigré who had been successful in various businesses including furs, real estate, and a large retail store. He and Mildred retired to Sun City in 1980, and loved it. And they stayed active. Aside from recreational activities they sat on half a dozen local and national boards and committees, from the United Jewish Federation to the Sun Health Research Foundation. They gave away money to various causes. They were respectable, admirable members of the community in every way. But they also enjoyed life. The good life was not something they had to strive for any more. It was all around them. And it was now – or never. When Max thought aloud about buying a local store he thought could make more money, Mildred told him,

* All patients and relatives referred to in this book are pseudonymous.

'Max, forget about it. I don't want to have the richest husband in the cemetery.'

Mildred was with her golfing friends one day, in about 1988, approaching a green on Briarwood golf course. She chipped up with the others, parked the cart, and walked out on to the green. When it was her turn to putt, she stood before her ball, reached down with her club—

What's Mildred doing? the others wondered. They stared at her, then at each other. Mildred's ball was well inside the green, yet Mildred was tapping it with a nine iron, instead of a putter.

The incident passed, but Mildred's golfing friends came to see it as the start of something. Something going wrong. Mildred was only in her early seventies, but they all knew almost anything could happen at that age. In the Sun Cities, it was almost like an old-fashioned plague was around. It could hit anyone, at any time. Your heart went. Or you got the cancer. Or things went wrong with your mind.

As the months passed, and similar incidents occurred, her friends noted sadly that Mildred played golf less and less, and then not at all. No one had the nerve to mention it to Max.

One day, at home with Max, Mildred asked, 'Max, will you drive me to the beauty salon?'

Max thought that was odd. Mildred always drove herself to the beauty salon. 'The car's in the garage, honey.'

'I know.' She sounded irritated. 'Max, I can't find the clutch.'

Can't find the clutch? To Max, that was a curious thing for her to say. She had never had problems driving before. But he drove her to the beauty salon anyway. Mildred was a strong-willed woman. It was almost always better not to argue with her. She was almost always right, anyway.

Max himself, it should be said, was not a weak-willed man. He had had an extraordinary life, living and fighting through two world wars, the first as a child in Byelorussia – kidnapped briefly by thieving Cossacks – and the second as a US Army sergeant. After World War II he had become a multi-millionaire, and had made it look easy. Max was a man who got things done.

Still, it took years for Max to admit to himself that something was wrong with Mildred. It took years of being confronted with subtle, then bizarre changes in the wife he had known and loved for half a century.

Mildred stopped driving altogether. Then walking became a problem; she began to get lost. One day she came out of the ladies' locker-room at Briarwood after a swim and began wandering aimlessly in the parking lot. 'I was just walking home,' she indignantly told Max when he caught up with her in the car.

She found it harder to explain to Max when one afternoon she wandered down the street from their home, through the unlocked front door of a neighbour they did not even know, and into the living-room. 'Mr Weller, I'm sorry to bother you . . .' the telephone call began. Everyone but Max and Mildred seemed to know what was happening.

Mildred began to accuse Max of speaking too harshly to her: 'You're not nice any more,' she would tell him. She walked out of a Jewish Federation benefit concert that she herself had helped to arrange, complaining that the music was too loud. Though never jealous before, she falsely accused Max of having a mistress.

And then there were the headaches. 'Oh, Max, my head hurts,' she would say. For that, Max finally brought her to a neurologist. He now feared the worst: Alzheimer's disease, a slow burn of dementia. Personality changes and memory loss were the obvious symptoms; possibly headaches were another sign.

The neurologist sent Mildred for a CT-scan, a detailed three-dimensional probe of her brain using computer-guided X-rays. The results came back. 'Good news,' said the neurologist. 'Mildred has had a series of small strokes in her brain. It's not serious. A couple of aspirins a day should take care of the headaches.' Mildred took the aspirins, and the headaches went away. But her personality continued to change.

Around October 1990, as they drove home to Sun City from a summer on the relatively cool California coast, Mildred turned to Max and began to complain once again, out of the blue, that he had become unbearable to her. She insisted that he stop the car. She wanted to get out, right there on the interstate, and walk home. Max persuaded her to stay. But he decided it was time to bring Mildred to the neurologist again.

Max Weller was a wealthy man, and as a donor to many causes, not least medical ones, he had considerable sway over doctors. These doctors promised him they would keep these first visits off the record. One neurologist, at the Mayo Clinic in Minnesota, assured Max that he had actually hidden Mildred's file at his home, in case a careless secretary at the office saw it and sent it out somewhere. It was important to Max that people not have cause to whisper: 'Mildred Weller is being tested for Alzheimer's.'

But of course, Mildred Weller was being tested for Alzheimer's.

Testing for Alzheimer's in a living person had never been an easy task, and even in the early 1990s it was something neurologists found difficult. The distinctive kind of brain-cell damage caused by the disease was not routinely detectable by CT-scans, MRIs, EEGs, or other diagnostic techniques. And despite breathless press-releases by scientists who claimed to have found telltale protein markers of Alzheimer's in patients' blood or cerebrospinal fluid, no such tests had been accurate enough to enter commercial use. Alzheimer's could really only be confirmed by the same method its discoverer, Alois Alzheimer, had used in 1906: looking directly at a sample of brain tissue under a microscope. In theory, one could get such tissue from a living patient by doing a brain biopsy. But what person wants a doctor to drill a hole in her skull and draw tissue out of her live brain with a large syringe? In practice, Alzheimer's was only confirmed after death, at autopsy.

While the patient was still alive, neurologists could still do a few things. They could establish, using IQ and mental status tests – 'spell bright backwards,' 'OK, now count down from one hundred by sevens' – that the patient suffered from dementia. They also could try to rule out the alternative causes for this dementia, usually leaving in the end only the most common and most hopeless cause: Alzheimer's.

The neurologists in Mildred's case chased down the three usual alternatives. They found that her problem, in the end, was not really a stroke, or stroke-related haemorrhaging. And there was no significant narrowing of arteries that fed her brain. And there was no cancerous tumour causing damage inside her brain.

That left Alzheimer's. The problem was, when the neurologists gave Mildred the IQ-type tests, to confirm dementia, they found a curious thing. She still scored high enough to seem, by American medical standards, *compos mentis*. In other words, she was such an intelligent woman that despite mental deterioration painfully obvious to those who knew her she remained clearer-headed, on the prescribed tests, than many 'normal' people her age. The neurologists threw up their hands. By the book, by objective diagnostic measures, they could not diagnose Mildred Weller with Alzheimer's.

To some of the neurologists working on the Weller case, this must have come as a relief. A diagnosis of Alzheimer's was all pain, and no gain. A diagnosis would not enable Mildred to qualify for drug treatments, because there were no drug treatments for Alzheimer's. It was an incurable, terminal disease.

After two more excruciating years, with further and more rapid mental and physical collapse, Mildred Weller was finally diagnosed with probable Alzheimer's. By that time, early 1992, the disease had eaten away at the networks in her cortex, her emotion-controlling amygdala and hippocampus and other limbic structures, and she had almost completely lost the personality that her husband knew as 'Mildred'. She no longer could walk without assistance. Soon she would not be able to feed herself successfully, and would also lose control of her bladder and bowels. She was simply forgetting how to do all these things. She was unlearning them as she passed down through mental adolescence and childhood to a sullen, barren infancy. What one neurologist has called 'an eight year death sentence' was now well under way.

Max put Mildred in the best nursing home in Sun City. He visited her two or three times each day. He played music: Glenn Miller, Tchaikovsky, Beethoven. He brought in her piano, together with the piano bench whose seat-cushion she had once expertly embroidered. He touched her and soothed her and reassured her of his presence. He made himself aware of virtually every detail of her daily rhythm, and made sure the nurses did their jobs right. And though he knew that there was no official treatment for Alzheimer's, approved by the Food and Drug Administration, he went out and sought the most promising experimental treatment he could find.

Which brought him, almost immediately, to a neuroscientist named Joe Rogers.

2

Brain 204

Even as he drifted up from the warm depths of sleep, Joe Rogers knew who had caused his telephone to ring at this ungodly hour. He managed to get the receiver off the hook and bring it over to his ear.

Doctor Rogers? asked the late-shift operator at Boswell Hospital.

Rogers grunted and felt around on the night table for a pad and pencil. As he did so he noticed the time on the electronic clock. Two a.m. Right in the middle of the night. Why were the dead so inconsiderate?

Doctor Rogers, the operator went on, I've just had a call from Nurse Marley over at Camelot Nursing Home. Sir, she asked me to tell you that Mr Edgar Morton has passed away.

Rogers thanked the operator, hung up, and dialled the nursing home. Nurse Marley told him what had happened. Mr Morton had died in his sleep, at some time between twelve-thirty and one-thirty. The physician on call that night had just been in to formally pronounce Mr Morton dead.

Rogers got dressed and went out to his car. It was a cool night. Back inside the house, Rogers's wife and children were warmly asleep.

Joe Rogers never questioned the value of his work, yet there were times when he wondered whether he was getting too old for these wee-hour activities. He was physically fit; he jogged every day, and played golf with an enviable handicap of just two strokes. Still, there was no getting round the fact that he was fifty and one-half years of age. His hair was almost entirely grey. Imagine blending together – morphing, as they say in Hollywood – the actor Larry Hagman with his short grey hair and white moustache and J R -Texas-oilman drawl, and television mogul Ted Turner with his short grey hair and white moustache and Georgia-good-old-boy drawl. The result would be someone looking and drawling just like Rogers, who was from Mississippi.

Rogers gunned the car engine and left his quiet suburban home of Spanish-tile-and-stucco behind. Soon he was out on the 101 loop freeway heading south for Sun City. At this hour it was only a six-minute drive to the two small buildings of the Sun Health Research Institute.

After parking on the street outside, Rogers opened the front door of the Institute's two-storey administrative building, jogged up the stairs to his secretary's office, and opened the cabinet containing his patient files.

Jacobs . . . Johnson . . . Jones . . . Kalstrom . . . Lennert . . . Maringo . . . Morton—

He took out the Morton file. Edgar J. Morton, seventy-eight years of age, wife deceased, had been diagnosed with Alzheimer's about five years before. The course of his disease had been fairly ordinary. There were no 'flags' in the file, warning Rogers to take special precautions in handling Mr Morton's brain. There was no evidence that the brain, which Rogers soon would hold in his very hands, had been destroyed by anything other than Alzheimer's disease.

The file noted that the Menke Funeral Home and Mortuary Service would be taking care of Mr Morton's mortal remains. Rogers called the Menke twenty-four-hour answering service, and left a message asking someone from the funeral home to go over and take Morton's body from the Camelot Nursing Home to the Boswell Hospital morgue. Neither the local funeral parlours nor the nursing homes would have cooperated with such late-night requests unless they had long acquaintance with Joe Rogers and his research. They knew it was in a good cause.

With the body on the way, Rogers telephoned the four others on his team. In half an hour they all met, more or less wide awake now, at the three-storey building next door where the Institute's laboratories were housed. They drank coffee and began suiting up in blue operating-room gowns.

As it is with scientific research in the United States, the team was composed largely of highly educated immigrants: Libuse Brachova, a neuroscientist from the Czech Republic, specialized in cell culture techniques. Lucia Sue, an American of Chinese descent by way of

Trinidad, headed the Institute's autopsy programme. Lih–Fen Lue, a slim Taiwanese woman, and Scott Webster, a tall Californian who at this hour badly needed a shave, would oversee the neuroscientific analyses of the tissue that was recovered.

Dressed now in their gowns, the five Alzheimer's researchers walked out of the laboratory building and across an empty street to the back lot of Boswell Hospital. Lucia Sue wheeled a cart with a white plastic bucket full of cold saline solution. Scott Webster lugged a briefcase full of surgical instruments. They could have made use of the instruments already available at Boswell, but Rogers didn't like to impose on the pathologists there any more than necessary.

They went in through a back door, down a hallway and through a series of interior doors into a refrigerated room, where Lucia Sue left the cold saline bucket. Then they opened a second door in the refrigerated room, and entered the morgue. There was no basement at Boswell. The morgue was on the ground floor.

They turned on the lights. Bright lights. The autopsy table lay in the centre of the room, a gleaming *tabula rasa* of stainless steel. The team members put on latex gloves – one pair, then another over it. They arrayed their surgical instruments on a white cloth on a wheeled tray next to the autopsy table.

Five or ten minutes after the researchers had arrived, the Menke black hearse pulled up at the hospital's back entrance. The driver, a young man wearing a dress shirt and dark trousers, opened the back and slowly rolled out a special wheeled, extendable metal gurney. On the gurney, beneath a white sheet, was a body. He wheeled it into the hospital and through the corridors, until he had reached the morgue. He greeted Rogers and the others, who thanked him for taking this trouble. No problem, he said. Glad to help. Then he went back outside to the front seat of his hearse, to listen to late-night talk radio, and maybe have some cigarettes. He'd have the body back before long. It would be a little lighter.

Rogers and the others lifted the body from the gurney on to the autopsy table. Then Rogers peeled back the sheet. Edgar James Morton was still wearing the nursing-home pyjamas he had died in. His eyes were closed. His face was gaunt and vacant. Death had taken him by stages, slowly, until for the last year he had lain in a foetal position, fed intravenously, with no more control over his bodily functions, and no greater consciousness, than a foetus has.

It was now about three-thirty, by the prominent wall clock in the morgue. Rogers and the others put on blue surgical caps that covered hair and ears, and blue surgical masks for their mouths. To keep bone chips and tissue fragments out of their eyes, they put on special facemasks made of clear, curved plexiglass that extended down to their chests. Somewhat like the kind arc welders use.

Rogers called for a cardiac needle. When it was handed to him, he punched it firmly into Mr Morton's chest, through thin membranes and withered muscles, to a depth that meant it had penetrated the heart. Rogers pulled back on the plunger to fill the large syringe tube with blood.

When he had collected as much as he could, and had handed the syringe to one of the others, he proceeded quickly to the next step. He took a scalpel and pressed its point into the skin above Mr Morton's right ear, feeling it sink through the soft skin, all the way to the skull. Holding the blade against the hardness of the skull, and holding up Mr Morton's head with his free hand, Rogers pulled the scalpel through the skin around the back of the head, until it came to the left ear. There was little blood.

Rogers now grasped the upper edge of the incision with one gloved hand, holding it open while he reached in with the scalpel and began cutting away pieces of connective tissue between scalp and skull. He pulled upwards on the increasingly loose scalp as he continued to probe and cut, 'teasing it open' with the scalpel. It was as if Mr Morton were wearing a whole-head mask, or a large toupee, and Rogers were now slowly pulling it off, from the back of his head to the front.

After a few minutes of this, the scalp had been pulled and stretched forward so far that it lay, inside out, across Mr Morton's face, hanging down from a line above the eyes. The top of Mr Morton's skull was completely exposed. Rogers put away the scalpel, and picked up the electric bone saw.

The saw, known also as a Stryker saw, had a semi–circular serrated blade about the size of a halved silver dollar. The blade did not rotate or spin. It vibrated a distance of merely one–eighth of an inch back and forth, but at a speed of hundreds of cycles per second. It was the same kind of saw used to cut open plaster casts when broken arms or legs had healed. It was preferred because it was so extraordinarily safe. Human skin or tissue was flexible enough that, in contact with the vibrating blade, it would simply vibrate along with it. But bone or any other hard material would be rapidly cut.

The saw whirred loudly and bone dust now flew out from the table against Rogers's mask and gown as he cut around the top of Mr Morton's skull. He proceeded in a seven-inch-diameter circuit above the ears and across the forehead. In the middle of the forehead he turned the blade and made a short zig-zag, to ensure snug and proper replacement of the skull cap later. When the skull cap had been cut through all the way around, Rogers took a stainless-steel instrument that looked like a miniature crowbar. He inserted it into the groove cut by the saw, just above the left ear, and twisted it lightly. There was a muffled, liquid popping noise, and the skull cap came off. Rogers placed it on the table.

Light grey membranes glistened across the top of the brain, packaging each hemisphere. Scott Webster reached in and spread the hemispheres with his hands, while Lih-Fen Lue took a spinal needle, inserted it down between the hemispheres and into the top of the spinal column, and sucked out a sample of cerebrospinal fluid.

Rogers now regarded the brain. There was no 'gross pathology', which is to say, no obvious damage. The characteristic lesions of Alzheimer's would be clear enough when the sectioned brain was later stained and put under a microscope. But at first glance with the naked eye, it didn't look too bad, only a little withered. Alzheimer's disease moderately shrunk the brain.

Rogers looked for evidence of strokes, but found none. Many old people had had strokes before dying. Strokes were blockages of blood vessels that killed brain areas by starving them of oxygen. Old strokes were normally evident as brown areas of deadness within the brain. As long as they didn't cover too wide an area, Rogers could cope with those old strokes. Recent strokes were another matter. If Nurse Marley at Camelot Nursing Home had informed Rogers that Mr Morton had died of a stroke, Rogers would have thanked her for calling, hung up the phone, and returned swiftly to sleep. Killer strokes could turn the brain literally to mush. When one popped open the skull cap on a person who had died of a big stroke, the brain would often just ooze right out on to the table. The stroke destruction, even if it didn't affect the entire brain at first, stimulated a massive clean-up effort by immune-system scavenger cells which pumped out large amounts of neuron-killing chemicals in an effort to break down and digest all the deadness. Beyond a certain amount of destruction, there was just no way the brain was going to recover. So strokes were bad news. Rogers knew there could be worse news: tiny holes all over the brain, which under a microscope made the brain look like a variety of Swiss cheese. That could be Creutzfeldt-Jacob Disease, rare but also 100 per cent fatal, and contagious. CJD's cause hadn't been absolutely established* but whatever caused it was unusually resistant to sterilization techniques. CJD also was seldom evident from a quick glance at autopsy, which was one of the reasons Rogers always checked his files first. If the patient had declined very rapidly, with signs of muscle incoordination, Rogers had to suspect CJD and take extra protective measures in the morgue.

Three-fifty. Rogers reached in between the skull and the brain, holding them apart with the fingers of one hand, while with the other he began scalpelling away the brain's various connections to the rest of the body: facial nerves, auditory nerves, optical nerves. Then he began working his way down the front of the brain, pulling back the brain from the front of the skull and cutting away the cranial nerves and arteries there until he could see the brain stem and spinal cord. Holding the brain back with one hand, he reached down with the scalpel, as far down as he could, and sliced cleanly through the upper spinal cord.

The brain was now essentially free of its body. Rogers put aside the scalpel, took the brain with both hands, and pulled gently, easing it back and forth until it popped out whole. He placed it on a nearby scale, let it settle, and Lucia Sue wrote down the number of ounces it weighed. Libuse Brachova snipped a small sample of tissue from the neocortex, the higher brain function region, and placed it in one of her cell culture dishes. She then capped the dish, removed her facemask and surgical mask, and walked with the dish back to the lab. Meanwhile Rogers took the brain again and placed it, without splashing, in the bucket of cold saline. Lucia Sue put a plastic lid on the bucket, placed a sheet over the lid, and wheeled the bucket

---

* The current theory is that CJD and related diseases (BSE, Scrapie, kuru) are caused by a mutated, oddly-folded version of a normal brain protein. When it comes into contact with normal versions of the protein, this mutant form can induce them to fold in the same odd way. This 'domino effect' results in widespread brain damage because the mutant form of the protein is effectively toxic to neurons.

back out of the hospital. Following Brachova, she crossed the street
to the laboratory building. No one stopped her to ask what she had
in the bucket.

While Brachova began work on her cell cultures, and Sue started
the long process of cutting the brain into sections and preserving
them for laboratory study, Rogers, Lih-Fen Lue and Scott Webster
quickly finished up in the morgue. Rogers cut Mr Morton's pituitary
gland from an area inside the skull just above the mouth, and
removed the nearby trigeminal nucleus, a terminal for the nerves
that controlled facial muscles. He had promised to send as many
trigeminal nuclei as he could to a colleague at the Wistar Institute in
Philadelphia. In fact, samples from brains like Mr Morton's were sent
by Rogers's lab to dozens of other researchers around the US. Rogers
would usually get something in return, such as a special, hard-to-find
laboratory reagent, or even a small funding grant if the recipient was
a commercial laboratory.

Four o'clock. Time to close up. To reduce the likelihood that
spinal fluid would seep out of the head, Rogers, Lue and Webster
packed the inside of the skull with wadded-up paper towels. Then
Rogers placed the skull cap back on the lower skull, snugly matching
zig-zag notch to zig-zag notch. When the skull was in place again,
he pulled the scalp back over it tightly. He placed a few sutures along
the original incision on the back of the head, and stepped back to
admire his handiwork. When Mr Morton was cleaned up, dressed in
his best Sunday clothes, and properly presented in a casket, none of
his mourners – except the relatives who had signed the consent forms
– would know that he had already donated his brain to science.

Rogers, Lue and Webster picked up the body again, and placed it
on the gurney. Then they began peeling off their masks and gloves,
washing up. The man from Menke's, alerted by the departure of
Brachova and Sue, emerged from his hearse, came to get the
body, and wheeled it away to store in a refrigerated room at the
funeral home.

The three neuroscientists washed off the autopsy table using hoses
of hot water and a strong antimicrobial solution known as Amphyll.
When the table was clean, they mopped the floor. They rinsed their
instruments, sterilized them, put them away in the suitcase again,
and walked across to the lab. It was still dark outside.

On one wing of the second floor of the lab, the brain was already proceeding along a kind of assembly line, a series of holding and cutting and freezing instruments arrayed across one long surface against the north wall. Here the brain was being cut into dozens of 'slabs' the thickness of thin-sliced bread. The slabs from the left hemisphere would be preserved in a kind of anti-freeze solution at minus 20 degrees Centigrade. They would be used for direct inspections of the brain by microscope. The slabs from the right hemisphere, to be used for molecular biological analyses, would be flash-frozen and stored in a special freezer at minus 80 degrees Centigrade.

The more quickly the samples were preserved, the more useful they would be for research. American Alzheimer's scientists who collected human brains for their research averaged six hours from time of death to autopsy. Six hours meant a lot of tissue deterioration. Rogers, with his extraordinary concentration of Alzheimer's patients here in the Sun Cities, averaged three hours. It was hard to see how it could be done much faster.

After talking to the others for a while, Rogers went over to the Institute's administrative building, which contained his office and, during work hours, a small support staff. Through the window he could see Scott Webster come out of the lab and place a white box by the door. It contained some of Mr Morton's blood and spinal fluid samples, now packed in special containers. In a couple of hours, a courier from a local clinical analysis lab would come to collect them.

Rogers remained in his office, working on papers he was writing, answering mail, signing administrative letters. He chatted on the phone with fellow scientists, and Institute benefactors, and relatives of patients. He walked to the lab several times, to talk with Brachova and Webster and the others. Around noon he drove home through bright hot sunshine, had lunch with his wife, and went to sleep. Rogers did not keep count in his head, but the recovery of Mr Morton's brain had been the 204th such operation his laboratory team had performed.

3

Inflammation

A lot of people in Sun City knew Joe Rogers. They knew him as the nice neuroscientist who came to their church group meeting, or Rotary or Lions' Club meeting, or square dance club meeting, and asked them please to donate their brains to him. 'Rats and cats and dogs don't get Alzheimer's,' they had all heard him say. 'Only humans get Alzheimer's. And that's why we need human brains for our research.'

Rogers was the nice neuroscientist who also patiently explained that he needed not just the brains of people with Alzheimer's – in any moderately-sized audience in Sun City, there would be at least several relatives of Alzheimer's victims – but also brains from people who had died of other causes, to enable comparisons to be made. With his Mississippian cadence, Rogers would assure his audience that the bodies of donors would not be disfigured; they could have an open casket. And for those whose religious beliefs left them . . . uncertain . . . about the ramifications of having no brain in the afterlife, Rogers would gently tease: 'You might think that St Peter won't let you in without a brain, but the thing is, he might be so impressed by what you did, that he'll let you in anyway.' Rogers further promised all donors of non-Alzheimer's brains that when they died their relatives would receive from him an official letter outlining the results of his laboratory's examination of the brain – Rogers would smile at this point in his monologue – 'And I'll tell them you were right all along: there was absolutely nothing wrong with your brain.' And the grey-headed Rotarians and square dancers and church group members would laugh and slap their thighs, and somehow, the idea of actually signing the paperwork and donating their brains would become a little more conceivable.

What had never really been conceivable, throughout the long, sad history of Alzheimer's research, was that those brains could be kept free from dementia, in later life, with a simple, inexpensive and already-available class of drugs: anti-inflammatory drugs such as ibuprofen and indomethacin. But that was what Joe Rogers had been saying to the scientific community: Alzheimer's disease inflames the brain. It drives the local immune system into a frenzy, releasing harmful chemicals that damage innocent cells, thereby doing to one's neurons more or less what arthritis does to one's joints.

This was, to say the least, an unconventional hypothesis. Small wonder that it had come from Rogers, a man who – had the chips fallen a bit differently – would never have been a scientist.

He had grown up in Oxford, Mississippi, where his father, Joseph Sr, was a prominent physician and for a time the head of the state medical association. A man who cast a shadow. Joe Jr felt pressure early on to become a doctor. But Oxford was Faulkner country, and he wanted to be a writer instead. Or a golfer. One of his best friends was the son of the pro at the local club, and most every day the two boys played a round there, getting better and better, Rogers's handicap falling steadily till it reached the low single digits. But at Emory University in Atlanta, where Rogers matriculated in 1963, there was no golf team. He took his BA degree in English literature, and also, grudgingly, took the courses in chemistry and biology that he needed to go to medical school. Rogers was a headstrong boy – smart, cocky – but when it came time to decide what to do with himself, post-graduation, his father's pressure won out. Young Joe applied and was accepted to the medical school of the University of Mississippi, 'Ole Miss'. His father was proud of him.

Something inside Rogers – some drop of rebel blood – didn't accept this state of affairs. After Christmas in his second year at Ole Miss he drove to Atlanta to see his girlfriend. He told her he wasn't sure he wanted to be a doctor. He wasn't sure he wanted to be on the career treadmill already. Just rolling along towards doctoring, and saying, 'Say ahhhh', and playing golf on Wednesdays. The golf part he didn't mind. He was nearly good enough now to play professionally. No, it was the doctoring part that bothered him. He wanted to really live, to experience the world, to roam around and have adventures and write about them. Some of this thinking had been inspired by an old college friend whom Rogers arranged to meet while he was there in Atlanta. The friend was just about to run off to the Bahamas, to fish and swim and laze about and live the Huck Finn life. As Rogers listened to his friend's stories about what he was going to do out there in the Bahamas, and how he could keep the good times rolling more or less indefinitely, the Huck Finn life started sounding pretty good. The day his friend flew out to the Bahamas, Rogers sold his car in Atlanta, got all his money out of the bank, and took the next plane he could to Nassau.

Three weeks and a few adventures later, the pooled resources of the two young men had dwindled to where it would buy them each a one-way flight to Miami, with ten cents left over for a local phone call. So they flew to Miami and they spent the dime calling another friend, whose folks owned an old hotel. It was a flop-house type of place by the looks of it, but they gratefully stayed there for a few days, and Rogers looked for work, and eventually he found a job as a copyboy with the *Miami Herald*, making coffee for the reporters, and tearing wire service stories off the ticker machines and putting them on the proper desks. Meanwhile, back in Mississippi, medical school classes had resumed. Joe Rogers, former student, was quickly being forgotten. In the household of Rogers Sr he was *persona non grata*.

A month or so after Joe Rogers had joined the *Herald* there was a teacher's strike in Miami. With his English lit. degree, Rogers managed to get a part-time job as a strike-breaking substitute teacher. He wrote up a piece about what it was like to be a strike-breaker, a scab, there inside the embattled Miami school system. The *Herald* ran the piece and promoted him to the obituary pages, and allowed him to branch-out into occasional feature stories. One was about a local man with no legs who had built a personal gyro-copter for himself. After six months with the paper, Rogers was made a staff writer on the city desk, covering the local crime and police beat. Meanwhile, in his spare time, he was writing the novel he had always wanted to write. The big one. It was about a young man, growing up in Mississippi in the fifties and sixties. In the shadow of a successful, staid father. The novel slowly grew and grew, as Rogers worked in Miami, then served a stint with the Mississippi National Guard, and eventually made his way back east to a better-paying job in Atlanta. There he worked as a copywriter for an ad agency. One of his clients was the manufacturer of an ointment for chapped cow teats.

*   *   *

Well, the novel went the way of most novels, into the wastebasket, and Rogers began to wonder whether leaving medical school had been such a good idea. Had he stayed, he would be finishing his residency somewhere. Perhaps he would be a budding surgeon. In any case, it was now too late.

Over one or two dark nights in Atlanta, fuelled by Gallo Hearty Burgundy and his usual brash confidence that he could do just about anything if he set his mind to it, Rogers decided that he would become . . . a neuroscientist. Neuroscience was new, and hot, and it attacked the biggest conundrum in science: the human brain. Why the hell not?

Rogers saved his money, started sending out applications, and eventually landed a place in the neuroscience PhD programme at the University of California at San Diego. Four years later – now married, with two kids – he started a postdoctoral fellowship at the nearby Salk Institute, in the laboratory of the famous neuroscientist Floyd Bloom. There he realized he had a problem. It started with itching around the eyes and a runny nose, whenever he was in the room where the lab animals were housed. Eventually he began sneezing violently, and having asthma-like breathing difficulties. By 1982 he had to wear a gas-mask device with a heavy filter to protect him from the animal hairs and other airborne rat and guinea-pig and dog and pig debris that were inflaming his immune system. Without the mask he could spend no more than a few minutes in the animal room before becoming incapacitated by asthma-like symptoms. Rogers knew that this situation couldn't last. He began to ask himself: What biomedical research can I do that will be scientifically important, yet will not involve working with laboratory animals?

Rats and cats and dogs don't get Alzheimer's . . .

Rogers decided to go with Alzheimer's research, which by the early 1980s had become very interesting. Scientists had begun to recognize that the disease was much more widespread than previously thought. It now seemed to account for the majority of cases of what had been ignored for years as mere 'senility'. That put it near the top of the list of leading killers of Americans, behind such monsters as vascular disease (heart attacks, strokes) and cancer. The challenging thing about Alzheimer's was that it seemed more closely associated with the ageing process than any other big disease out there. About 4 per cent of seventy-five-year-olds had it, and the incidence rose to 20 per cent at age eighty, and more than 30 per cent at eighty-five. If one lived beyond ninety it would probably be unusual *not* to have Alzheimer's. So the battle against Alzheimer's would be a battle against one of the great, seemingly inexorable processes of human mortality.

Alzheimer's had been considered a 'small' disease for so long because its rarer form was described first. People thought it was all there was.

The rare form was described by Professor Alois Alzheimer at a meeting of German psychiatrists in Tübingen in early November 1906. Alzheimer presented the strange case of Frau Auguste D, who had died in a Frankfurt mental asylum the previous April. Alzheimer noted that she had suffered from severe, slowly progressive dementia over the previous five years. After her death, Alzheimer had taken samples of her brain tissue, had stained them with a silver-based compound often used for such analyses, and had put them under his microscope. Through the microscope he had observed two unusual features that seemed to be associated with the woman's dementia.

The first were 'plaques', small regions of diseased and dying neurons, throughout certain regions of Frau D's brain. At the centre of each plaque was a clump of some kind of insoluble protein. Proteins that accumulated in such insoluble clumps had been found in other diseases, and had been given the general term 'amyloids', from the Latin word *amylum*, for 'starch'.

Even in some areas where there were no amyloid plaques, Alzheimer noted the presence of strange tangles of some unknown fibril-like substance. They curled like mattress-springs within neurons, or protruded from obviously dying neurons, or simply lay in the empty zone of death where neurons had once been. These came to be known as 'neurofibrillary tangles'.

Alzheimer had seen amyloid plaques in brains from non-demented patients, especially older ones. They seemed to be a normal part of ageing. He also had seen the strange tangles in the brain of a person who had died in 1898 of 'progressive paralysis'. But in Frau Auguste D's brain there were many more plaques than he usually saw, and he had never seen them together with the neurofibrillary tangles.

What was more, Frau D when she died had been only fifty-one years old.

Special relativity was invented, and general relativity, and the quantum theory, and the laser. And scientists designed a bomb that could level a large city. And men walked in space and cavorted on the moon. And robot ships landed on Mars, and flew past Saturn.

And still almost nothing was added to the store of knowledge about Alzheimer's disease. Only in the mid 1970s was it widely recognized that senile dementia was simply a more common and later-onset form of the rare disease Alois Alzheimer had described. Only then did senility begin to be seen as unnatural, unacceptable – an illness that could be treated, and perhaps one day eliminated altogether.

The rare form of the disease that Alois Alzheimer had described was hereditary. It ran in families. And that gave scientists studying Alzheimer's a potential advantage. If they could find the mutated gene responsible for the rare, early-onset form of the disease, they might also be able to understand the common, later-onset form of the disease. It seemed likely that the same process was occurring in both, but was speeded up, for genetic reasons, in the rare form. It was like cholesterol in atherosclerosis: some people for genetic reasons accumulated cholesterol plaques in their arteries quite rapidly, while for most people the process occurred only slowly. Either way, the problem was the accumulation of cholesterol, and the solution was to reduce the accumulation. Perhaps a similar solution would come out of the study of Alzheimer's.

But looking into the genes of early-onset Alzheimer's patients wasn't that simple. Trying to find a malfunctioning gene in a human genome made of tens of thousands of genes was even harder than looking for the proverbial needle in a haystack. One had to look at people with the rare, highly genetic form of Alzheimer's, and then compare their genes to those of healthy relatives, sorting through the many genetic differences one would expect anyway, until the right gene was found. Even with the sophisticated molecular biological techniques available now, in the present, at the turn of the millennium, that is a difficult, expensive, time-devouring task. In the 1970s it was out of reach. Most of the progress in those years had to come from direct studies of the autopsied brains of Alzheimer's victims.

One of the things that was obvious about Alzheimer's disease was that it affected the 'higher' brain functions of memory and reasoning and personality, leaving intact such 'lower' functions as breathing and heartbeat. The destruction caused by Alzheimer's was reminiscent of that scene in the film *2001: A Space Odyssey*, where the astronaut removes the higher memory cards from the amok super-computer 'Hal' – and as he does, Hal's thoughts collapse down to his earliest, most childish memories, until his personality is extinguished and he is left with only automatic unconscious life-support functions.

Unsurprisingly, neuroscientists looking at Alzheimer's brains found that most or all of the deathly plaques and tangles occurred in the parts of the brain that controlled higher functions, such as the neocortex (memory and logical reasoning) and hippocampus (emotion and spatial reasoning). But in the late 1970s they began to find evidence that only a certain type of neuron in these regions was affected by Alzheimer's.

These were years when neuroscientists were just beginning to grasp the basic fact that neurons communicated with each other using a complex system of chemicals known as neurotransmitters. When a neuron sent a signal to another neuron, it caused chemical changes to occur down the length of one of its 'axons' – long tendrils reaching out to other neurons – until the proper chemical neurotransmitter surged like a spark from the end of the axon into the space (the 'synapse') between the axon terminal and another neuron's axon terminal. The neurotransmitter that had been spat out into the synapse then caused chemical reactions in the other axon, and those fired along the long arm of that axon to its governing neuron, which then fired neurotransmitters down other axons, towards other neurons, and so on. Somehow all this sparking and spraying of neurotransmitters added up to sentience, to intelligent action, to consciousness.

At that time in the 1970s there was much attention to another common neurodegenerative disease associated with ageing: Parkinson's disease, which involved a progressive rigidity and tremor in certain muscles. Neuroscientists had found that Parkinson's seemed to be caused by the destruction of a small brain region called the substantia nigra, which normally supplied a neurotransmitter called dopamine to other areas. Pharmaceutical companies wasted no time looking for ways to artificially boost dopamine levels, to make up for the loss.

They went on to make a drug, Levodopa, that was metabolized to dopamine in the brain and, when given to patients, clearly delayed the progress of Parkinson's. Naturally, scientists looked for a similar mechanism, and a similar solution, in Alzheimer's disease.

Well, seek and ye shall find. Scientists knew that a drug called scopolamine reduced memory and attention-span when given to rats, monkeys, and people. They also knew that scopolamine interfered with the workings of a neurotransmitter called acetylcholine. Thus they reasoned, correctly, that acetylcholine was important to memory and attention-span. They then took a leap and guessed that acetylcholine was to Alzheimer's what dopamine was to Parkinson's: a vital stuff that was lacking, and had to be resupplied artificially.

In pursuit of evidence for this hypothesis, neuroscientists began looking at the brains of Alzheimer's victims, comparing them with 'healthy' brains to see if there were any differences in the amounts of acetylcholine, or in the numbers of acetylcholine-sensitive neurons. They knew they could find the acetylcholine neurons, for example, by using radioisotope-tagged antibodies that fastened tightly to neuron acetylcholine receptors. All they had to do was pour the antibodies on a slice of brain, rinse lightly, and then put photographic film on top to record where the radiation-emitting isotopes were still clinging.

Suddenly, the field of Alzheimer's research came alive. Starting with an article in the *Lancet* in 1976, 'Selective loss of central cholinergic neurons in Alzheimer's disease', paper after paper was published showing that Alzheimer's brains, compared to normal brains, suffered from severe depletions of acetylcholine-associated neurons.

A massive herd of scientists now gathered, and began to gallop in the direction of acetylcholine. From cramped university lab benches staffed by a single sleepy postdoctoral student, to gleaming laboratories at well-funded research institutes and pharmaceutical companies, researchers aimed to repeat the Parkinson's story with acetylcholine and Alzheimer's. They feverishly studied the acetylcholine system, and they looked for ways to boost acetylcholine levels in the brains of people with Alzheimer's.

One of the most respected Alzheimer's researchers in those days was Professor David Drachman at the University of Massachussetts. New researchers and new grant money were flowing into his lab, and papers on Alzheimer's were steadily flowing out. Joe Rogers, looking for a good Alzheimer's lab in which to work, approached Drachman in 1982 and asked if he could come to U-Mass. Drachman was impressed by Rogers's research at the Scripps Institute, and eventually agreed.

So Rogers and his family moved 3,000 miles east–north–east, to cold Worcester, Massachussetts. Rogers became an assistant professor of neurology, and began to perform studies on the brains of humans who had died of Alzheimer's. He became responsible for collecting many of those brains: driving his little Mazda hatchback out to distant hospital morgues in the dead of night, over frosted country roads, donning scrubs alone and painstakingly cutting open scalps, sawing open skulls, and returning before dawn with a full bucket sloshing next to him in the passenger footwell.

After a few years spent characterizing the ravages of plaques and tangles in these brains, Rogers began to lose interest in what he was doing. He began to test Professor Drachman's patience and tolerance. The young, unknown, but cocky neuroscientist made clear to the older, very-well-known neuroscientist that he didn't believe in following the acetylcholine herd any more. He didn't agree with the direction most of the U-Mass research was going. In fact, he was beginning to think that virtually all the scientists out there doing Alzheimer's research were wrong about the disease.

Even when he had been at the Salk Institute, Joe Rogers had had reason to question all the emphasis on acetylcholine. In one project, which eventually resulted in a paper in *Nature*, he and other Salk researchers had shown that the levels of another neurotransmitter, called somatostatin, were also reduced in Alzheimer's brains. That meant acetylcholine wasn't the only answer. By the time he had been at U-Mass a couple of years, Rogers's scepticism about acetylcholine had grown enough that he decided to make an abrupt change in the direction of his work.

It was a good time for a change in direction. Thanks in part to the availability of better laboratory reagents, scientists were beginning to glimpse the fact that neurons of many types, across the neocortex and hippocampus and limbic areas of Alzheimer's brains, were dying in substantial numbers. And it wasn't because some mysterious drop in acetylcholine or any other neurotransmitter

had starved them. It wasn't that the brain merely needed a boost
with a neurotransmitter-enhancing drug. No, the neurons were
being killed by something that had nothing to do with a lack of
acetylcholine. The fall in acetylcholine was completely secondary
to the loss of cells. It was a result, not a cause. It was the silence
after a massacre. The solution, it was becoming clear, was to stop
the massacre, to block whatever it was that was killing the neurons.
Force-feeding the remaining neurons with acetylcholine was like
shouting at a man in a coma, to try to wake him up. Much better
to fix whatever it was that had brought him so close to death.

The herd that had gathered in pursuit of acetylcholine would
begin to break up around the edges in the mid 1980s, although its
core would still carry enormous momentum. Drug companies would
continue to push acetylcholine-boosting drugs through their R&D
pipelines. Science journalists would continue to cover press releases
issued by the acetylcholine camp, and would continue to accept, even
into the 1990s, that Alzheimer's was 'caused by abnormalities in the
brain's chemical messenger system'. And hundreds of neuroscientific
careers, fuelled by long-term grant money, would continue to run
their dead-end course, everyone pretending not to see what an
enormous mistake had been made.

Some time in late 1984, Joe Rogers was sitting in his office at U–Mass.
It was wintertime, and cold. There was snow outside. He hated cold
and snow.

He was in one of those funks, like the one that had gripped him
in Atlanta more than a decade before. It wasn't that he wanted to
abandon science, or even Alzheimer's research. He just needed
something definite to aim at. Something to keep him interested.
Something no one else was doing.

He cleaned off his blackboard and began to write down all the
things that, as far as he knew, could conceivably be killing cells in
the brains of Alzheimer's patients. For each one he asked himself:
'Is this really something I should be pursuing?'

Acetylcholine? No. Acetylcholine was the bandwagon everyone else
was on.

Neurofibrillary tangles? These were the tangles of fibrils seen inside
many of the neurons of Alzheimer's brains. Obviously they should
be looked at. Perhaps some malfunction in the brain was causing

the NFTs to form inside neurons, and the NFTs were then slowly killing the neurons. But NFTs were found in a number of other brain diseases, and could be the result of neuronal decay, rather than the cause. Also, Rogers knew of other researchers, with more resources and grant money at their disposal, who were already looking at NFTs. Rogers didn't want to be part of that herd either.

Amyloid? This was the insoluble, clumped protein found at the centre of the amyloid plaques in Alzheimer's brains. Clearly, amyloid was a major suspect. Some thought that it was just a by-product of the disease process, but Rogers considered it a worthwhile target for investigation. Perhaps the amyloid was deposited abnormally, and then became toxic to neurons. But again, too many people were already looking at this, and they were better equipped to do so. There was George Glenner, a biochemist and an expert on other conditions – 'amyloidoses' – where insoluble clumps of protein were deposited in the body. Glenner had just published the protein sequence of the amyloid clumps found in Alzheimer's, dubbing the short protein 'beta amyloid' for the 'beta-pleated' shape it took. There was also a scientist at Harvard about Roger's age, a neurologist named Dennis Selkoe who was looked upon as a whiz kid. He had been researching NFTs, but now he was turning to beta amyloid.

Aluminium deposition? Researchers were beginning to talk about the possibility that toxic levels of aluminium, perhaps from tinfoil or dissolved in the water supply, were accumulating in brain cells and causing Alzheimer's. This was an especially popular idea among the general public, where people believed in the presence of invisible, slowly lethal and deforming environmental toxins almost as fervently as they had believed in invisible demonic influences a few centuries before. Respected researchers had even reported finding evidence of abnormal amounts of aluminium in Alzheimer's brains. Rogers considered the aluminium hypothesis a reasonable one, but he guessed that if aluminium was the cause, there would be a lot more Alzheimer's than there already was. Aluminium was everywhere. In any case, Rogers knew that other researchers, such as Dan Perl at the University of Vermont, were way ahead in this area.

Slow or latent viruses? Now here was an attractive possibility. And it seemed that almost nobody was working on it. Yet it was well known that there were viruses out there that could linger in their host cells – including neurons – for years and years, only intermittently 'breaking out' and killing their hosts. Some of the herpes viruses were like that. There were herpes viruses that could somehow infect the trigeminal nerves inside the face, causing episodes of sharp facial pain. Perhaps an unknown type of herpes virus was infecting brains, and people became more susceptible to it as they grew older. Perhaps a genetic defect could make people susceptible to it at a younger age.

Rogers would spend the next three years looking for viruses in the brains of people with Alzheimer's. And after all this work he would conclude that his virus hypothesis had been wrong. When all was said and done – when all the red herrings and false trails had been left behind – he would find no viruses in Alzheimer's brains that were associated with the disease. Along the way, however, he would find something unexpected and interesting. He would find that, while there didn't seem to be any viruses in and around the plaques and tangles of Alzheimer's, there was something in there that had stirred up the immune system. Within the lesions of Alzheimer's, little immunological storms were raging.

In normal immune reactions, in parts of the body separate from the brain, a molecule called HLA-DR was usually expressed on the surfaces of some immune cells. HLA-DR was something like a battle-flag, hoisted aloft by immune cells to chemically rally the troops. Rogers and his colleagues got hold of a monoclonal antibody that specifically bound to HLA-DR. Using a solution of the antibody as their detector (the antibodies were labelled with a special chemically reactive dye) the team looked for evidence of HLA-DR in samples of Alzheimer's brains, as compared to control brains.

When Rogers saw the resulting images of the Alzheimer's and control samples, he was shocked. There was no significant evidence of HLA-DR on the control samples. But the Alzheimer's samples were clearly full of cells expressing HLA-DR. The HLA-DR molecules were being expressed by microglial cells and astrocytes, normally thought of as 'housekeeping' cells within the brain, useful for cleaning up debris.

Rogers knew it was possible that all these cells were in battle mode because they were busy breaking down and cleaning up dead neurons. But it was also possible that the cells were running amok on their own and causing direct harm to neurons. That was more or less what happened in the disease known as multiple sclerosis, though in that case the damage was done by T cells that had come in from the bloodstream and invaded the brain, attacking and destroying muscle-controlling neurons – mistaking friendly cells for foes. In this case the damage seemed to be caused by the microglial cells and astrocytes, locally based cousins of T cells.

Whatever was causing all this activity, the intense HLA-DR expression in Alzheimer's brain tissue was something no one had noted before. The brain was normally thought of as an immunologically 'privileged' area of the body, where raucous immune system battles almost never occurred. Alzheimer's scientists would now have to take these new findings into account.

Rogers wrote up his team's results into a brief paper, titled 'Neurovirologic and neuroimmunologic considerations in Alzheimer's disease'. He started sending it out to journals.

And . . . the paper kept coming back. Rejected by journal referees. The idea that the immune system itself was to blame for killing neurons was certainly an original idea. But that was the problem. It was too original. It just didn't seem credible to those who had been following, and advocating that others follow, more promising paths. Such as the acetylcholine path.

Referees were often older researchers who had been around the field longer. Ideally their job was to spot specific problems in the procedures reported in a scientific paper, not to dispute the paper's conclusions out of prejudice. But they were only human. They were a kind of self-reinforcing old boys' network. If they all felt like ignoring something, there was really no one who could overrule them. In rare cases, where it was clear that sheer bias was at work, a free-thinking journal editor would do so. But in most cases the journal editor was part of the same old boys' network and had the same prejudices.

Rogers reacted with anger when he saw what was happening. What to him was a significant piece of data was effectively being censored. What the hell were the old boys afraid of?

4

Voices in the Wilderness

Rogers went to Washington DC in the summer of 1986, to the annual Society for Neuroscience conference, and presented his data in the form of a 'poster' – a series of pages, with text and diagrams and photographs, posted on a wall or standing partition alongside other researchers' work. No referee could stop him from doing that. At large meetings there was always a part of a room set aside for such posters. Researchers could browse through the poster area, stopping to read the ones that interested them, perhaps also questioning the scientists who had written them.

Rogers watched with dismay as hundreds of researchers glanced momentarily at his poster, then walked past. Only one stopped to look. He was a postdoctoral researcher from a laboratory at the University of British Columbia in Vancouver. Rogers didn't know him. The young postdoc read through Rogers's paper, asked a few questions, then moved on.

In the months following the conference Rogers did further experiments. He went after other markers of immune activation – HLA-DQ, HLA-DP – and kept finding them in the plaques and tangles of Alzheimer's patients. The immune system was running hot in Alzheimer's lesions, and maybe was a big part of the problem. But no one out there was interested. Rogers seemed to be slipping out of the mainstream of Alzheimer's research, perhaps for ever.

Some time late that year, Rogers was contacted by a group of philanthropists in Sun City, Arizona. They, and the non-profit group that ran the Sun City hospitals, wanted to set up a non-profit institute for the study of Alzheimer's disease, and they were looking for a neuroscientist to head up the project. Rogers sent the group his c.v., went down to Sun City for an interview, and got the job.

Before he left, he stopped by a Sun City real estate office. He opened the glass door, walked into the office, and stood there waiting for someone to help him. He watched as people glanced up, then looked away as if he was not completely visible. They continued the various tasks they had been doing. What was happening here? wondered Rogers. Didn't anyone want to sell him a house? Eventually someone patiently explained that, regardless of the good work he might be doing for Sun City residents, he could not actually live in Sun City. He was only forty years old – way too young.

Rogers eventually found a house in nearby Glendale, and he moved there with his wife Mimi and their son and daughter. Aside from everything else, Rogers was glad to be back in a warm climate. He loved playing golf, and in southern Arizona one could do so virtually year-round.

The institute he now headed was supposed to be called the Institute for Biogerontology. That was a mouthful, and it sounded impressive. But it wasn't the same as being at a university. In fact, the institute at first was merely a vacant office in a vacant building near Boswell Hospital. Saying 'the Institute of Biogerontology' really only meant 'a neuroscientist from Mississippi named Joe Rogers'. It was essentially up to him to find the staff he would need, plus the money to pay them, plus the money to build a laboratory. In addition to all that, he knew he needed to start a brain-donation programme, so he could have tissue upon which to perform research. That meant he had to go around to Sun City church groups, square dance groups, the Lions' Club, the Rotary Club, and so forth, to make his pitch about brain donations. And when the consent forms were signed, and consenting people died, he would have to perform brain-removal autopsies at whatever hour of day or night they were needed. Rogers also needed a board-certified pathologist, to look over the brain samples he had removed, and to declare whether or not they met the criteria for Alzheimer's disease. Board-certified pathologists cost money.

Despite all these hassles and worries, Rogers liked being where he was. He liked being in control. As time went on and his fund-raising efforts paid off and the money started to come in, he began to spend his days designing the Institute's new buildings. His friend Max Weller, a great believer in delegation, would later say with an exasperated, heavenward glance that 'Joe likes to hammer in every nail'.

The one nail he couldn't drive home was the HLA-DR paper. He was increasingly convinced that the immune system activation in Alzheimer's brains had something to do – perhaps everything to do – with the killing of neurons. Immune cells when sufficiently enraged were capable of releasing powerful chemicals that could pop nearby cells like so many balloons. Even if the activated immune cells in Alzheimer's brains were supposed to be playing a clean-up role, getting rid of dead neurons, it was possible that they also were killing innocent bystander neurons. And Rogers had the data to support that possibility. But he couldn't get it published. Months, then years went by, and still it went nowhere. Finally, in 1988, Rogers managed to get a short paper accepted by the journal *Neuroscience Letters*. The paper was simply titled 'Immune system associated antigens expressed by cells of the human central nervous system'. That year Rogers got a similar paper, 'Immune actions in the nervous system – a brief review with special emphasis on Alzheimer's disease', into the journal *Drug Development Research*. And after a certain amount of 'begging', as he would later put it, he convinced the editor of *Neurobiology of Aging* to publish his original, albeit updated paper, now titled, 'Expression of immune system associated antigens by cells of the human central nervous system: relationship to the pathology of Alzheimer's disease'.

But it was too late. Well before any of these papers appeared, another paper appeared in *Neuroscience Letters*, titled, 'Reactive microglia in patients with senile dementia of the Alzheimer type are positive for the histocompatibility protein HLA-DR'. The lead author on that paper was Patrick McGeer, a veteran neurologist at the University of British Columbia. It had been one of McGeer's postdoctoral students who had read Rogers's poster at the Society of Neuroscience conference. Rogers, exasperated at being beaten to publication after all these years, suspected that McGeer's postdoc had simply noted his data from the poster, and had replicated his experiments. What really burned him was that the McGeer paper did not even reference his. Even if McGeer and his people had thought up the HLA-DR experiment themselves, he thought, they should have made note of his earlier work.

In the summer of 1988 there was a select gathering of Alzheimer's researchers at Cold Spring Harbor Laboratories on Long Island Sound. Rogers could see that most of the hottest researchers had been invited. Dennis Selkoe was there from Harvard, to talk about beta amyloid, already shaping up to be one of the most important focuses of research. Peter St George-Hyslop, also from Harvard, and Allen Roses from Duke University were there to talk about the genetics of familial Alzheimer's. Dan Perl, now at Mount Sinai Medical School in New York, was there to talk about aluminium. And Pat McGeer from Vancouver was there, to talk about his work on HLA-DR and microglial cells.

The chair of the conference was the venerable neurologist and gerontologist, Caleb 'Tuck' Finch, from the University of Southern California. Finch knew Rogers from way back and invited him to come and talk about his own HLA-DR results. Unfortunately, Rogers was placed after McGeer in the schedule, making it look once again as if McGeer's lab had been the first to do such work. When he finally got his chance to speak, Rogers referred eight times to 'Rogers et al 1986', the obscure abstract of his original HLA-DR paper that had been published in the Society for Neuroscience conference proceedings. He mentioned that some of his data 'have recently been replicated by McGeer and colleagues'. But McGeer's paper didn't reference Rogers's earlier work at all.

One evening after dinner Rogers walked out of the campus cafeteria and saw McGeer strolling on the sidewalk outside the building, casually taking the sea air. McGeer was a handsome, amiable-looking man, with a shock of black hair and a bow-legged gait from chronic tennis playing on the grass court he had at home. He looked as if he didn't have a care in the world. By contrast, Rogers's anger was starting to pump. Now was the time to confront the man. He went over to McGeer and, trying to sound relaxed, greeted him and shook hands, and then—

'You know, I was sort of – pissed off – to see you publishing my data like that.'

'Oh?' said McGeer, who appeared genuinely shocked. He explained that he had been working on the virus hypothesis for quite some time, since 1984 in fact, and after failing to find viruses had looked for immune system antigens as an indirect sign of some kind of viral infection in the brain. His postdoc had seen Roger's results on the poster, but both he and McGeer by then had disagreed with Rogers's suggestion that viruses were to blame. In any case, he had waited and waited for Rogers to publish those results but after two years had not seen them in print anywhere. So he had been unable to reference them when he published his own data. He was surprised that Rogers hadn't published first. And he was very sorry he had annoyed Rogers by publishing.

As McGeer went on, Rogers found himself more and more embarrassed that he had said anything. McGeer seemed like a genial, honest, decent fellow. Rogers realized that, angry as he had been, he could put this thing behind him.

By the end of the Cold Spring Harbor meeting, Rogers and McGeer had agreed to collaborate in their research. Rogers could see that he and the Canadian were very much in the minority in the Alzheimer's world. They had to hang together, as the old saying goes, or else they would hang separately.

Pat McGeer was one of those individuals who seem to possess, beneath a calm exterior, an unnatural abundance of energy – or vital stuff, or life force, or whatever one wants to call it. He was extraordinarily active, productive, and versatile. An all-rounder. As a young man at the University of British Columbia he had been the star forward for the UBC Thunderbirds basketball team. Fifty years later he would still remember the winter's day in 1946 when the Harlem Globetrotters had come to town: the line of fans a quarter mile long; the students climbing on to the campus coliseum to look down on the court from broken windowpanes in the roof; the Globetrotters' surprise at the skill of the young Thunderbirds; the legendary 'Trotters' manager Abe Saperstein yelling at his players at half-time, threatening to fine them, anything, they weren't supposed to be losing to these college kids; but the 'Trotters still losing to the Thunderbirds, 42–38, the crowd cheering, delirious, swarming on to the court, the UBC high scorer that handsome fleetfooted fast-dribbling 5ft 11 inch sophomore forward, Pat McGeer, who a couple of years later, just before entering medical school, would play for the Canadian team in the 1948 Olympics in London.

McGeer was later part of the first expedition to capture a killer whale, a creature then thought to be a bloodthirsty man-eater. He ventured to the Canadian Arctic in search of the fabled narwhal. He directed the Vancouver Aquarium. He served on the boards of several large corporations. He was an advocate for the use of methane as an alternative to gasoline fuels, and edited a book, *Methane, Fuel for the Future*. He was a member of British Columbia's provincial legislature for twenty-four years, ten of them spent in important cabinet posts for education and science. He wrote another book about that, titled *Politics in Paradise*. Throughout this time he also earned an MD in neurology and a PhD in physical chemistry, headed UBC's Kinsmen Laboratory of Neurological Research, and was an author on more than 200 medical research papers, plus two scientific books – one, the ambitious *Molecular Neurobiology of the Mammalian Brain*, with Sir John Eccles and McGeer's own wife, Edith, a neuroscientist herself. And somehow despite all this frenetic activity McGeer managed to look almost paranormally young. When Rogers met him he was already sixty-one, yet he looked the same age as Rogers, who was almost two decades younger.

The McGeer and Rogers collaboration was almost immediately fruitful. Their evolving hypothesis about Alzheimer's – that immune activity was contributing to the deaths of healthy neurons – had given them an advantage of sorts because it could be checked by simply looking around at people who already took drugs, anti-inflammatory drugs, to reduce immune activity in their bodies. If such people showed a lower incidence of Alzheimer's, that would suggest the anti-inflammatory drugs had done the trick, and that in turn would support the notion that inflammatory processes were at work in the disease.

Unknown to both Rogers and McGeer, four London physicians already had written a letter to the *British Journal of Rheumatology* in 1988, noting that patients with Alzheimer's disease had an unusually low incidence of rheumatoid arthritis. Of ninety-six patients the physicians had seen with Alzheimer's, only two also had rheumatoid arthritis, compared to twelve patients with rheumatoid arthritis in an age-matched control group of similar size. The London physicians, believing that having Alzheimer's protected one against developing arthritis, had speculated that there might be a genetic relationship.

Rogers and McGeer interpreted such data differently. To them, the data showed that anti-inflammatory drugs – which most of the arthritis patients would have been taking – protected against Alzheimer's by damping the immune system.

The two scientists quickly performed their own study, using hospital data from Sun City and various cities in Canada, and came up with even stronger evidence. Among Alzheimer's cases they found almost no cases of arthritis, and among arthritis cases they found almost no cases of Alzheimer's. Moreover when they scrutinized the records of patients who had both diseases they almost always found that either (1) the Alzheimer's dementia had developed long after the patient had stopped taking anti-inflammatory drugs, or (2) the arthritis had developed when the patient already had dementia.

Looking backwards at hospital records – a 'retrospective study' in the vernacular of medical science – was not the ideal way to conduct research. Data gathered that way had to be treated with caution until they were confirmed by 'prospective', forward-looking clinical trials, in this case trials of anti-inflammatory drugs in Alzheimer's patients. But the retrospective data Rogers and McGeer uncovered were so one-sided they cried out for attention. They suggested that the long-term use of anti-inflammatory drugs drastically reduced the possibility of getting Alzheimer's. And so far there were no treatments for Alzheimer's. And in the United States alone, there were 4 million Alzheimer's victims.

Further evidence for the inflammation hypothesis came from an unlikely source: a leper colony on the Japanese island of Nagashima. A Japanese physician who had visited the colony mentioned to McGeer at a conference that the leprosy patients there had an oddly low incidence of Alzheimer's. He speculated that because the leper colony was such a close-knit community, the elderly people there were kept more mentally active than usual, and their additional brain activity made them more resistant to Alzheimer's. McGeer, of course, looked for another explanation. He didn't see Alzheimer's as a disease that could be remedied by increased social interaction. He saw it as an organic process of brain-matter decay. He wanted to know what drugs the leprosy patients were taking.

Most of them, it turned out, were taking a drug called dapsone, the leprosy antibacterial of choice in Japan. McGeer grabbed his medical books and started reading about dapsone. And there it was: dapsone, according to the medical books, also had a strong anti-inflammatory effect. In earlier years it had been widely prescribed for rheumatoid arthritis and other immune disorders.

McGeer and a set of Japanese colleagues now went to work

studying Japanese leprosy patients. There were about 4,000 in all. How many of them had dementia? How many of those were still taking dapsone? The answer was that the ones still taking dapsone had about half the incidence of dementia of those not taking dapsone. And for those who had only been taking dapsone intermittently, the incidence of dementia was somewhere in between. That was a key piece of evidence, for it suggested a 'dose response effect'. In other words, the chances of dementia seemed to go down the more frequently one took dapsone.

McGeer and Rogers buttressed these findings with their own studies of autopsied brains from dementia patients. They noted that, out of some 169 consecutive brains studied by their groups in Sun City and Vancouver, none of the brains with typical Alzheimer's lesions was from a patient who had been taking anti-inflammatory drugs. None!

Around this time a group of Japanese researchers, alerted to McGeer's and Rogers's work, reported their analysis of sixteen autopsied brains from elderly leprosy patients who had been taking dapsone. In these dapsone-soaked brains there were not even any amyloid plaques. That was very surprising. Even non-demented elderly people normally have some amyloid plaques. The data suggested that the dapsone hadn't worked by merely reducing the damage caused in Alzheimer's. No, the dapsone apparently had worked by cutting off Alzheimer's at the source, by stopping whatever deep, ageing-related process actually gave rise to Alzheimer's in the first place.

The response to all this sensational data – data that illuminated a new avenue of research for desperately-needed anti-Alzheimer's therapies – was almost complete silence. The average newspaper reader or TV-watcher did not see any of it. In the popular consciousness of Alzheimer's research the inflammation hypothesis did not exist. Even among Alzheimer's scientists themselves, there was little response.

More than a year after McGeer's and Rogers's Canadian and Sun City data appeared in a letter to the British medical journal the *Lancet*, a group of researchers from the Mayo Clinic in Minnesota sent their own letter to the *Lancet*. Citing the McGeer and Rogers letter, they reported that they had looked at a large Mayo Clinic database. Among arthritis patients in the database, most of whom had at some point been prescribed aspirin or other non-steroidal anti-inflammatory drugs, there seemed to be a normal number who also developed Alzheimer's. Of course, they hadn't checked on the actual frequency of anti-inflammatory drug use among the Alzheimer's cases, but their findings generally seemed to contradict McGeer and Rogers's findings.

For Alzheimer's researchers already convinced by some other hypothesis, the Mayo Clinic letter would probably have been seen as sufficient reason to ignore McGeer's and Rogers's data. But the letters section of the *Lancet* was a relatively obscure place anyway, and probably few Alzheimer's researchers read either letter. In fact most researchers were probably not aware of any of McGeer and Rogers's data, because none of those data had been published in prominent places. The dapsone study had been published in *Dementia*, a journal with a tiny circulation that was largely among researchers outside the USA. The Japanese analysis of brains from dapsone-treated patients had been another *Lancet* letter.

Rogers and McGeer naturally tried to get their work published more prominently, in such journals as *Science* and *Nature*. But they had no success. At *Science*, they believed, the group of reviewers for Alzheimer's papers was a particularly entrenched group of old boys. To them the idea that some inflammatory process caused Alzheimer's apparently was too wild even to consider. There was also the fact that McGeer was out in western Canada, an emeritus moving into his mid-sixties, and upstart Rogers was down in the deserts of Arizona running a tiny institute nobody had heard of. Rogers watched as paper after paper, by researchers at Harvard and other big universities, was waved through by the old boys at *Science*. Some of those papers, for example by beta amyloid researcher Dennis Selkoe, represented excellent work. But others, as Rogers saw it, were just garbage; they seemed to have been published merely because their authors had an affiliation with a big university. The Harvard bias, Rogers started to call it. The Harvard old boys, protecting their own.

At Alzheimer's research conferences now, there was increasingly an atmosphere of resentment and antagonism. After the demise of the acetylcholine hypothesis the community for the most part had separated into two groups. The dominant group, the ones who had the media and the Harvard old boys on their side, were the proponents of the beta amyloid hypothesis. McGeer dubbed them the 'Baptists' – taking the 'Bapt' from Beta Amyloid ProTein. The second largest group were the 'Tauists'. Tau was the name of the protein that was the largest constituent of the neurofibrillary tangles. The Tauists believed that tau caused Alzheimer's. As a result, and to their great disgust, they too had largely been shut out from the pages of the big journals. And they were almost never mentioned in popular media accounts of Alzheimer's disease.

The connotation of Baptists and Tauists as competing religious groups was definitely intended by McGeer. He didn't have a name yet for the tiny cluster of immune hypothesis proponents. There were hardly any of them, anyway. Aside from McGeer's lab and Rogers's small lab, there were now really only two labs pushing the idea that immune factors were at work. One was led by Tuck Finch at USC, and the other by a Dutch researcher, Piet Eikelenboom. But the work published by those two was as obscure as McGeer's and Rogers's. While the beta amyloid bandwagon gathered momentum – as in years past the acetylcholine bandwagon had done – McGeer and Rogers could only watch in annoyance, sharing jokes about their predicament. McGeer kept returning to religious metaphors. The Baptists were 'false prophets', he said. By implication he and Rogers were the rightful prophets, rightful but ignored. They were voices crying in the wilderness.

But perhaps a day of reckoning would come.

5

The Harvard Bapist

Unfortunately for Rogers and McGeer, the idea of a day of reckoning, a day when the Baptists and their beta amyloid hypothesis would be swept from the field, was becoming increasingly difficult for most observers of the Alzheimer's community to imagine. The Baptists had a growing array of evidence on their side. And they had Dennis Selkoe.

Other scientists often found themselves in disagreement with Dennis Selkoe. They applied their own interpretation to the data coming out of his laboratory. But few suggested that his data were simply wrong, that Dennis Selkoe was a bad scientist, that the work he and his team had done was sloppy. In terms of intelligence, scientific integrity and attention to detail Selkoe seemed above reproach. Even non-Baptists admired him. Around 1986 a hotshot young venture capitalist named Kevin Kinsella began looking for a neuroscientist who would serve as chief consultant to his planned biotech company. The company would begin by trying to develop a treatment for so-far-untreatable Alzheimer's. Kinsella, who knew next to nothing about neuroscience, toured the Alzheimer's research community asking questions. He was a direct man, a plain speaker. One question he often asked was: 'Who is the best scientist in this field?' Kinsella asked Joe Rogers that question at a Society for Neuroscience conference and Rogers didn't hesitate. He said, 'Dennis Selkoe's your man.'

Inspired by a clever, charismatic woman who was his family's paediatrician, Dennis Selkoe had wanted to be a doctor from the age of about six. He wanted to be, and he was. He went to medical school at the University of Virginia, became a neurologist, and won praise from his patients. But even in his early years of medical school this fact confronted him: doctors were mired down in the trenches, fighting disease one patient at a time. They were only as good as the weapons scientists gave them.

And so, after finishing a postdoctoral neuroscience fellowship at Harvard in the late 1970s, Selkoe started a small research lab at the McLean Hospital, Harvard's psychiatric teaching hospital in the Boston suburb of Belmont. By then he had jumped, like many young neurologists and neuroscientists, into the high-stakes arena of Alzheimer's research.

The sandy haired, blue-eyed doctor – scientist made his name quickly. At the time many Alzheimer's researchers still believed that aluminium might have something to do with the disease. Some experiments had even shown that if one injected the brains of small mammals with aluminium, tangles like those seen in Alzheimer's would form in and around the mammals' neurons. Selkoe did his own experiment, injecting aluminium into the brains of about 100 rabbits. He found tangles all right, but they were not the neurofibrillary tangles seen in Alzheimer's. He published a paper on that, and lost interest in aluminium as a culprit in Alzheimer's.

By this time, 1981, a group of researchers led by Bob Terry at the Albert Einstein College of Medicine in New York had claimed to have isolated the protein that constituted most of the notorious neurofibrillary tangles. Terry and his colleagues had done this by taking samples of tangle-rich neurons, dissolving them with a standard solvent called SDS, and placing the resulting solution of proteins on a special slab of gel, using an electric field to separate the floating proteins by molecular weight. Comparing the proteins in a tangle-rich sample to those found in an ordinary sample, they found that one protein stuck out. The tangle-rich sample, but not the other, contained a protein with a molecular weight of 50 kilodaltons. Terry and his colleagues decided that this must be the mysterious protein that made up tangles.

There was a certain amount of celebration and congratulation over this result, for now the study of these inexplicable tangles could begin in earnest. Selkoe, however, had his doubts. He knew there was a filament-forming protein inside astrocytic cells that also had a molecular weight of 50 kilodaltons. When it came to taking samples of brain tissue for this kind of work, it was very hard to separate the astrocytic debris from the neuronal debris. So it was possible that the 50-kilodalton protein that the researchers had detected was simply this humdrum protein from the astrocytic cells.

Selkoe decided to do his own experiment. He prepared two gels, one with debris from tangle-rich neurons and one from ordinary neurons. He made sure the samples were extra pure to avoid contamination with astrocytic proteins.

And when he ran the gels he couldn't see any difference in the proteins that sorted out. There were no 50-kilodalton proteins in either sample.

So the 50-kilodalton proteins Bob Terry had found probably had been contaminants from the astrocytic cells. The problem was, Selkoe knew that one of the samples he had taken must have been full of tangles. Yet the two samples – one tangle-rich, the other tangle-free – looked identical when the electrophoresis gels were run. The proteins that jittered along the gel under the force of the electric field were all the same. So the question was: if the 50-kilodalton protein Terry had found was only a contaminant from astrocytic cells, then where had the tangle proteins been? On the gels there had been no evidence of them at all. Where the hell had they gone?

It eventually occurred to Selkoe that the tangled, helically twisted proteins might be so un-dissolvable that they had not even been digested by the powerful SDS solvent used before running the gel. He hypothesized that the tangle proteins, instead of mingling in soluble form with the other proteins, had been left behind, still clumped together, in the bottom of the test tube when the rest of the SDS-and-proteins solution had been squirted on to the gel. To check this hypothesis Selkoe collected the grainy insoluble residue that remained in the tube when everything else had dissolved into the SDS. Maybe, he thought, this insoluble residue was where the real tangle protein would be found.

Selkoe and his colleague Yasuo Ihara painstakingly prepared samples of this undissolved stuff, and mounted them upon special electron–microscope grids. If the stuff wouldn't dissolve for an electrophoresis gel, then maybe Selkoe could find it with a brute force method of detection: the electron microscope, capable of directly imaging even small proteins.

One hot July day at the McLean Hospital, Selkoe went down to the electron microscope lab and showered the pellet with electrons. If the microscope viewscreen showed evidence of the tangles, that would effectively prove his hypothesis.

The viewscreen showed an alien microworld of eerie, cathode-ray green, in which Selkoe saw, scattered about the distinctive tangles, paired helical fragments, like old mattress-springs in a junkyard. It was an exhilarating feeling. He knew he was in Alzheimer's research to stay. He published his results in *Science* and suddenly Bob Terry and the rest of the 50-kilodalton crowd had egg on their faces.

And some of them were no longer so friendly towards young Selkoe, but there wasn't much they could say. That was the thing about Selkoe. He could annoy you but there wasn't much you could criticize about him. He was meticulous, methodical. He was famous for his encyclopedic knowledge of the Alzheimer's field that he could articulate for hours on end with ease. He had spent a year in Germany during his teens and still sprinkled his conversation with German words whose meanings were just a bit more apt than their English counterparts. He had that Germanic aura about him of precision, of focus.

As it had been for aluminium, Selkoe lost interest in the tau protein and the tangles as potential causes of the disease. He reasoned that because the tangles were found in half a dozen other neurodegenerative diseases, they were probably part of a general response by neurons to certain kinds of damage. In Alzheimer's they seemed to appear only after the first thin clouds of beta amyloid had begun to form. They seemed more likely to be a result than a cause – more likely to be little molecular tombstones that neurons crafted for themselves as they lay dying.

Leaving tau behind, Selkoe turned his attention to beta amyloid. In 1984 he and his technician Carmela Abraham at the McLean Hospital narrowly missed being the first to isolate the protein and identify its protein sequence. The 42-amino-acid version of the protein they tried to sequence had a molecular grouping near one end that interrupted the sequencing process. The protein was thus 'blocked' and couldn't be fully sequenced. Amyloid expert George Glenner at the University of California at San Diego was fortunate to isolate slightly different, non-blocked amyloid from clumps in the walls of blood vessels around the brain. Glenner sequenced this amyloid, and published quickly in an obscure journal, and that was the end of that race.

In 1985 Selkoe moved his growing lab from the McLean Hospital to a building on the Brigham and Women's Hospital complex in Boston's Back Bay area, where he had done his neurology residency. This was Medicine Central – one of the most crowded conglomerations of hospitals and medical laboratories on the planet. With neuroscientist Howard Weiner, a renowned expert on multiple sclerosis, Selkoe formed the Center for Neurologic Diseases at Harvard in a set of laboratories overlooking Longwood Avenue.

The lab grew, and from Selkoe's end came paper after paper on beta amyloid. With a dozen researchers and technicians and more than a million dollars in annual funding, his lab was about the largest working on Alzheimer's. Through the consulting role he began in 1986 with Kevin Kinsella and his biotech company, San Francisco-based Athena Neuroscience, he also had a major influence and a big stake in the largest commercial lab studying the disease.

To both researchers and journalists Dennis Selkoe became increasingly well known not just as the head of a major laboratory but as an active evangelist for the beta amyloid hypothesis – a Baptist, as Pat McGeer would say. At conferences, in review papers, and over the phone with someone such as Gina Kolata of the *New York Times* or Jean Marx of *Science*'s research news section, he was eloquent and thorough in reciting the reasons one should believe in the beta amyloid hypothesis.

He liked to begin with this reason: beta amyloid deposition occurred first in the brain. It occurred in older people when they were still healthy, *compos mentis*. It occurred before the formation of tangles and before the killing of neurons. It occurred early and it progressed slowly and eventually – as the killing started – the diffuse, cloudy, 'cotton wool'-like deposits became denser and turned into rough, hard, insoluble nuggets of the stuff. Apparently somewhere in this densifying process the beta amyloid had passed some critical threshold and become toxic to neurons. If beta amyloid deposition was merely a result of the neuron-killing process, a tombstone like the neurofibrillary tangles, then it should appear only after neurons started to die – and clearly that wasn't the case.

In 1987 several labs reported cloning the gene responsible for beta amyloid. One of these labs was run by Konrad Beyreuther at the University of Köln. His group cloned the longest gene sequence and announced that beta amyloid came from a gene that coded for a large protein, 695-amino acids long. This large protein was soon dubbed 'APP', for 'amyloid precursor protein'. When APP was cleaved in a certain way, at two key points, presumably by enzymes, one of the resulting fragments was beta amyloid. Just what were the normal functions of APP and its daughter protein beta amyloid? Well, nobody really knew. Perhaps beta amyloid had no normal function. Perhaps it was cleaved from APP only under unusual circumstances, and only did harm to the brain. Or perhaps it had normal functions but, at too great a concentration – as for cholesterol – it became a bad thing.

To Selkoe and other Baptists, this was where the second big reason for believing in beta amyloid came in. When the gene for APP was cloned, researchers noted that it lay on human chromosome 21. For the Baptists that was exactly where it should have been. If the beta amyloid hypothesis was correct – that is, if the deposition of amyloid clumps in the brain resulted in the killing of brain cells – then any process that increased the production of APP in the brain (thus increasing the production of beta amyloid) should hasten the kind of neuronal damage seen in Alzheimer's disease. As the Baptists knew, there was a relatively common genetic disease that increased the production of APP by 50 per cent. It was a disease that resulted when, at conception, the original cells of a developing person each ended up with three copies of chromosome 21 instead of the normal two. The disease was known as Down's Syndrome.

In Down's Syndrome not just APP but all chromosome 21 proteins were overexpressed, leading to a host of problems. People with Down's Syndrome often died by the age of fifty. But well before then their brains would contain at least diffuse deposits of beta amyloid. It was hard to say how badly such people suffered from dementia because they were substantially mentally retarded to begin with, and died young, perhaps before a full–blown Alzheimer's-type disease could manifest. But it had always seemed a good possibility that Down's Syndrome and Alzheimer's were related, through some gene on chromosome 21. Now, with the discovery that APP was on chromosome 21, it seemed clearer what the relationship was.

The chromosome 21 discovery was quickly followed by another: a team led by Peter St George-Hyslop, Rudi Tanzi and Jim Gusella at a Harvard genetics lab reported that members of a family with the rare, early-onset form of Alzheimer's had defects somewhere on chromosome 21, apparently in the same neighbourhood as the APP gene. The suggestion was obvious: the defect probably changed the amount or structure of APP, which in turn boosted production of beta amyloid, which clumped in the brain at an abnormal rate and killed neurons and thereby caused Alzheimer's.

One of the missing links in the Baptists' profession of faith was, of course, the actually toxicity of beta amyloid. When you placed it in a laboratory dish with neurons, did it kill them? Put another way: the suspect (beta amyloid) might have been caught at the scene of the murder, but did he really possess a plausible murder weapon?

Labs were now able to produce beta amyloid at will instead of harvesting it from the brains of dead people. They could snap the genetic sequence of some or all of the beta amyloid region into a special culture of cells, and the cells would pump out this 'recombinant' beta amyloid. Now the race was to answer the question of beta amyloid's toxicity: to find the smoking gun.

Working with Dennis Selkoe, two researchers at the University of California at Irvine, Janet Whitson and her lab chief Carl Cotman, published the first report in this area in *Science* in 1989. They used what they had at the time, which was a 28-amino-acid fragment of recombinant beta amyloid. Adding it to cultures of neurons from the hippocampuses of rat brains, they watched to see if the neurons – which normally died steadily in culture dishes – would die at a faster rate when assaulted with the beta amyloid. But they found the opposite. The neurons stayed alive longer with beta amyloid. The stuff seemed to be healthy for them.

The Baptists had hardly had time to consider the ramifications of this strange result when *Science* published a new paper, this one by Bruce Yankner, whose lab was a few blocks away from Selkoe's on the campus of Children's Hospital. The title of Yankner's paper said it all: 'Neurotoxicity of a Fragment of the Amyloid Precursor Associated with Alzheimer's Disease'.

Yankner and his colleagues had inserted part of the APP gene into an immortalized, forever-dividing line of cells known as PC12 cells. The PC12 cells began expressing a fragment of APP that contained beta amyloid. The PC12 cells were then chemically induced to change into a neuronal type of cell. When they did, these 'neurons' that produced beta amyloid began to die.

Yankner and his team sought further proof. They took the beta amyloid soup produced by these cells, and ladled it into a culture of rat hippocampal neurons like the one Whitson, Cotman and Selkoe had used. The neurons getting the beta amyloid soup died quicker than neurons that didn't. When Yankner's team added anti-beta-amyloid antibodies to this mixture, to block beta amyloid's effects, the killing of neurons slowed.

Whitson, Cotman and Selkoe had been wrong, it seemed. But why? A year later, Yankner answered the question. Using a 40-amino-acid version of beta amyloid, Yankner and two colleagues added it to the usual rat hippocampal neuron culture. And just as Whitson, Cotman and Selkoe had found, Yankner too found that the beta amyloid was 'trophic', or life-preserving, for the neurons. But that was only when the neurons were in a still-developing, foetal-stage state. When they had become more mature and had started to extend little axons and dendrites – becoming more like the neurons in the brains of older humans – they reacted to the beta amyloid not by living longer but by dying faster. So beta amyloid was toxic after all. Hallelujah. And it was about time.

Yankner's reports of these results, delivered at conferences and in October 1990 in *Science*, had a grand and, it was said, pedantic tone to them. At the Society for Neuroscience meeting that summer he even finished his talk by paraphrasing a famous concluding line by Watson and Crick, the discoverers of the double-helix structure of DNA. Such flourishes seemed to convey the message that the big mystery of Alzheimer's had finally been solved. The other message seemed to be: Dennis Selkoe and his big-shot colleagues did sloppy work.

Selkoe literally could not take this sitting down. At conferences when Yankner would invite questions after a talk, Selkoe would stand up and question his Harvard colleague about his methods, and question and question, making clear that he thought the methodological sloppiness was coming from the other side of the podium.

Meanwhile, outside the conference rooms, in the media, everything seemed fine. Beta amyloid was toxic. It killed neurons. It deposited in neuron-killing clumps and caused Alzheimer's.

When the *Wall Street Journal* published Selkoe's comments on Yankner's results, there was no hint of a fierce dispute. 'It's the strongest evidence to date that the amyloid beta protein itself is directly driving the disease process,' said Selkoe. 'That's quite exciting.'

In fact, working with rat neurons in culture was only a small step towards demonstrating beta amyloid's role in Alzheimer's. Culturable rat neurons were very unlike elderly human neurons, which essentially could not be cultured. What the Baptists really needed, and wanted, to nail down the amyloid hypothesis was an experiment using a good, live animal model of the disease. The animal would be like the proverbial black box. Put in too much beta amyloid, and watch what came out. If what came out was Alzheimer's disease, with all the characteristic plaques and tangles, then almost certainly the beta amyloid had caused it. Even more importantly, such animals could then be used to study potential Alzheimer's therapies.

The problem was, rats and cats and dogs did not get Alzheimer's. Monkeys did seem to get Alzheimer's-like lesions if they lived long enough, but lab monkeys were far too expensive and too long-lived to do this kind of work in.

As genetic engineering techniques had advanced, it had become possible to create 'transgenic' mice – mice whose genes had been altered to overproduce a given protein. So far no one had developed a transgenic mouse that overexpressed APP and went on to develop brain plaques and tangles like those in Alzheimer's. There were mice that overexpressed APP, and some of them had a few amyloid deposits but not like those found in Alzheimer's patients. In those mice, for whatever reason, there wasn't the neuronal alteration seen in Alzheimer's.

Then suddenly lightning struck. In the fall of 1991 Dennis Selkoe received a package from the editors of *Nature*, asking him to write a commentary on a paper they intended to publish just before Christmas. The paper, whose lead author Shigeki Kawabata was employed by Yamanouchi Pharmaceutical Co. in Tokyo, was about a transgenic mouse strain that looked like the perfect model for Alzheimer's.

Kawabata, working out of a lab at Mount Sinai Medical School in New York, where he was on sabbatical, had inserted a human

APP gene in mice so that they overexpressed a fragment of APP like
the one Bruce Yankner had used in his latest toxicity experiments.
Kawabata had done this by injecting the embryos of lab mice with
copies of a fragment of the gene, and then breeding the resulting
mice until he isolated a line of mice that always overproduced the
human APP fragment in their neurons. As the little genetic mutants
grew up, Kawabata periodically sacrificed them and sent their brains
to Gerald Higgins, a researcher at a National Institute on Aging lab
in Baltimore. Higgins sliced up the brains and examined them for
evidence of Alzheimer's-type lesions.

What Higgins reported finding was astonishing. At four months
of age the mice already had the kind of diffuse beta amyloid deposits
seen in elderly humans. At eight months the mice's brains were
killing fields. There were amyloid plaques surrounded by dead cells,
and there were neurofibrillary tangles, and they were in the same
places – the cortex and the hippocampus – that one normally found
them in humans. Unfortunately for the poor mice, they seemed to
be a perfect, speeded-up model of Alzheimer's disease.

Selkoe wrote his one-and-a-half page commentary for *Nature*. He
expressed some doubts about the precise applicability of the mouse
model to human Alzheimer's, but in general his tone was confident.
The message one got, reading the commentary and the Kawabata
paper, was that beta amyloid could be a direct cause of the disease,
and as the mouse model suggested, probably was. Neurofibrillary
tangles were clearly secondary. Inflammation didn't even seem worth
mentioning any more.

And it now seemed that Alzheimer's research was turning a corner,
looking down one last stretch to the finish line. Transgenic mouse
models like the one Kawabata had developed could be cheaply
bred and licensed to laboratories worldwide. Any researcher who
thought he had a drug that blocked amyloid deposits could give
it to the mice to see if it really prevented their Alzheimer's-type
pathology. Research could shift from the basic science of the disease
to technologies for curing it.

Selkoe, who prided himself on his thoroughness, knew that there
were a few loose ends to all this. In fact it could have been argued that
aside from the Kawabata-Higgins mice the beta amyloid hypothesis
had been taking some serious blows.

For one thing, Selkoe still didn't understand why beta amyloid was not toxic to neurons in his lab while it was toxic to neurons in Bruce Yankner's lab a few blocks away. Other researchers were also trying to duplicate Yankner's results, but were having the same problem as Selkoe's team. They couldn't get the toxicity they wanted. Yankner in the summer of 1991 had announced finding Alzheimer's-like damage in mouse brains he had directly injected with beta amyloid. That had suggested an easy solution to the problem of animal models: just inject mice directly with amyloid. But Selkoe's lab, and others – including his allies at Athena Neuroscience – hadn't been able to duplicate the amyloid-injection work in monkeys. It was suggested that whatever damage there was in Yankner's mouse brains had been caused by the needle that injected the beta amyloid.

As sometimes happens when a researcher publishes a finding but others are persistently unable to reproduce it, tempers flared. It was widely believed that Yankner, whatever his data, was consistently overinterpreting those data. There was a spreading rancour around Yankner, like the neurological fire that raged around amyloid in Alzheimer's brains.

And clearly some of this rancour was coming from his main rival down the street. In the science media one report noted with polite imprecision that 'Yankner has been particularly challenged by investigators allied with Athena Neuroscience'. Well, Yankner was challenging them right back, hinting that his chief critics were simply angry that he had beaten them to the development of an animal model – hinting, in other words, that they had let concerns about big money slop up their own science.

The smoke hung heavy over Longwood Avenue, between Yankner's lab and Selkoe's.

To the Baptists' further dismay the genetic evidence also had taken a strange turn. It had finally been found that some early-onset Alzheimer's sufferers with chromosome 21 defects had mutations located in their APP genes, and that those mutations caused beta amyloid expression to be increased. But it also had been found that this chromosome 21 defect was very rare, even among people with early-onset Alzheimer's. Most early-onset cases, it was becoming clear, were caused by as yet unknown defects on chromosome 14, which in genomic terms was continents away from the APP gene.

For now the evidence from genetic studies no longer supported the beta amyloid hypothesis as it once had. The gene defects responsible for most early-onset Alzheimer's cases might turn out to cause immunological problems, or defects in the tau protein, instead of the over-production of beta amyloid. There was just no way to know without further, painstaking scientific work.

So. Loose ends. But with the Kawabata-Higgins transgenic mouse model now in existence, those loose ends seemed less important. The transgenic mice represented an elegant *in vivo* experiment showing, more clearly than any experiment yet, that beta amyloid was somehow the culprit.

One day, after the transgenic mouse paper was published, Selkoe telephoned Gerald Higgins down in Baltimore. Those transgenic mice were going to be geese that laid golden eggs, and Selkoe – like any foresighted Alzheimer's scientist – wanted in on the project. He wanted to run some of his own experiments with the mice. He suggested to Higgins that they collaborate.

Higgins agreed to consider doing some experiments with the distinguished Harvard researcher. And after two or three weeks in which Higgins delayed Selkoe, citing important ongoing work, he agreed to let him come down to his lab in Baltimore for a visit.

Selkoe arrived on a Monday morning, pulling up to the National Institute on Aging hospital complex by taxi from the airport. Higgins, a bearded man in his late thirties, greeted Selkoe warmly but seemed nervous, distracted.

What's wrong? asked Selkoe.

Higgins explained with shrugs, waves of the hands, that people were raising absurd questions about his work, about his photographs and his evaluations of the transgenic mouse brains. And he was sick and tired of it. He was ready to just walk away from the whole goddamn thing.

Wait a minute, said Selkoe. You have this beautiful transgenic model and you want to walk away from it? Why not stick to your guns?

Yeah, yeah, you're right, responded Higgins. But he remained nervous. Pursued by demons that Selkoe couldn't yet perceive.

As part of his visit Selkoe wanted to see the mouse brain tissue samples that Higgins had analysed for the *Nature* paper. There was a double-headed microscope in Higgins lab, and Higgins put a slide with a silver-stained tissue sample into the focal pit. Selkoe looked through one set of binocular lenses, and Higgins through the other. As his eyes focused, Selkoe immediately saw something wrong with the sample. In fact it looked not like one sample but like two samples, partly overlapping. The spacings of the cells were different, from one to the other, and the two even seemed to have been stained to slightly different hues, as if they had been prepared separately. Selkoe noticed that while one sample clearly had signs of Alzheimer's-type plaques and tangles, the other one clearly didn't. It was as if the first sample, with Alzheimer's-type lesions, was from a *human* brain, while only the normal-looking sample was from a mouse brain.

After a minute or so Selkoe said, Jerry, you know – what it really looks like here is that you have two pieces of tissue.

Oh, no. That's just a break in the tissue.

I don't think so. It really looks like two pieces of tissue.

What are you saying, Dennis? That's ridiculous.

I know it's absurd, Jerry, but that's what it looks like.

And Selkoe described the differences in the tissue in detail. But Higgins, growing angrier, stated that Selkoe was wrong, that what he was suggesting was offensive. The sample was perfectly normal. And the argument went on, getting hotter and hotter, as Selkoe refused to back down, and Higgins grew more agitated, searching the lab for another sample he said he had from the same diseased mouse brain. I'll show you, Dennis. I'll convince you. And frantically pulling out drawers. And not finding the other sample. And then:

You know what, Dennis? I just realized I sent them all up to Jon Gordon at Mount Sinai.

Yeah, but you would have kept some of them.

No, I sent them all. Jon will have them. And when I get them from him I'll show you.

Prodded by Selkoe, Higgins called Jon Gordon, the other author on the transgenic mouse paper, from there in the lab. Gordon told Higgins he hadn't received any tissue samples from him.

When that conversation was finished Selkoe turned to Higgins. Well, I hope you kept the airbill number from the Fed-Ex.

Higgins looked around some more. Jeez. I guess I lost the airbill number.

Soon it was time for Selkoe to go to a nearby building for a lecture he'd promised to deliver. He did the lecture, ate a quick lunch, and then came back to Higgins's lab. Higgins announced that after more rummaging around he'd found another slide with tissue from the mouse brain.

Selkoe looked in the microscope again. And again he saw two overlapping pieces of tissue. But this time he noticed that they were still floating in the preparation gel. The pyrex cover slip hadn't completely settled down on to the sample yet. As Selkoe immediately knew, that was because the sample was not one that had been lying around gathering dust, as Higgins claimed. Higgins obviously had just prepared it.

As the silver-stained tissue swam before Selkoe's eyes, the neurologist realized that the impossible had just become almost certain. The beautiful data that had made such a splash in *Nature*, in the Alzheimer's research community, and around the world's media, had all along been crudely faked. The 'Alzheimer's mouse' tissue had simply been an overlap of one piece of tissue from a healthy mouse and another from a human who had died of Alzheimer's. How Higgins thought he could have got away with it was the biggest mystery. It seemed completely irrational.

When it was time for Selkoe to go to the airport, Higgins walked him out of the building. On the way they had to pass along a glassed-in walkway to another building. At the end of the walkway was a door. Higgins tried to open it, but it was locked. He began shaking it, suddenly almost shouting – Goddamn it! Why the hell can't I get out of here?!

Selkoe pointed out that there was a card reader next to the door, and that Higgins had an ID card on a small chain around his neck that would open the door.

Oh yes. Of course.

A minute later Selkoe got into the waiting taxi, nodded at Higgins, and headed for the airport. What he would later call the 'most painful moment of my professional career' was over. He never saw Higgins again.

On the suggestion of Henry Wisniewski at the New York State Institute for Basic Research, the National Institute on Aging had already begun asking neuropathologists for their opinion on the mouse brain photographs published in *Nature*. There was general agreement that the images didn't look much like the brains of mice. Soon Kawabata and Gordon admitted that they could not reproduce the original findings in subsequent mice from Kawabata's amyloid-overexpressing transgenic line. They could find none of Higgins's plaques or tangles. The *Nature* paper, and the once-beautiful mouse model, was retracted. Then Gerald Higgins resigned from his laboratory and, as far as the scientific community was concerned, vanished into thin air.

6

Mac Attack

Strange and tragic it may have been, but the dissolution of Gerald Higgins's transgenic mouse model was a triumph for those opposed to the beta amyloid hypothesis.

Still, it left intact the central conundrum of beta amyloid: namely, that the protein seemed toxic to neurons in some labs, such as Bruce Yankner's, yet didn't seem toxic in other labs, such as Dennis Selkoe's.

At the same time it was obvious that beta amyloid was somehow connected to the disease process. Long before dementia became manifest the amyloid slowly began to assemble in the brain, in those fuzzy, unaggregated clouds. And later, when the patient had begun to lose his mind, the amyloid lay aggregated in hard, insoluble clumps, like fragments of a bomb at the centre of tremendous destruction. Beta amyloid's long presence at the scene of the crime had to be explained.

To Joe Rogers, the evidence of inflammation in and around the Alzheimer's plaques also had to be explained. And try as he might, he couldn't explain it.

In the early spring of 1991, Rogers was invited to a small gathering of scientists in San Diego. It was to be a symposium at which they would discuss the latest work on the inflammation hypothesis. Zaven Khachaturian, head of Alzheimer's research at the National Institute on Aging, had organized the meeting. So Rogers flew across the desert from Sun City to San Diego, with his golf clubs and lecture notes and a few slides, and at the appointed time stood at a podium and told everybody where he was in his research: at a dead end, more or less.

The immune system, he explained, had gone to battle mode in and around Alzheimer's lesions. Microglia, the immune system's chief representatives in the brain, clearly had their war paint on. But he and Pat McGeer didn't know why.

One of the clues he had hoped would bear fruit came from McGeer's laboratory. McGeer and his postdocs had found the lesions of Alzheimer's filled with a set of proteins known as complement.*

Complement proteins represented one of the most potent weapons in the immune system's arsenal. The complement system apparently had been designed by nature for a specific, simple purpose: to blow holes in diseased or otherwise unwanted cells.†

The complement attack started when an initial and otherwise harmless form of complement, known as C1, was produced by activated immune cells – including microglial cells – at the scene of an infection or some other immunological tempest. In such places there would often be antibodies pinned tightly to foreign proteins on bacteria, or to pieces of virus protruding from infected cells. When C1 encountered an antibody locked in embrace with its foreign foe, the out-hanging tail section of the antibody triggered a chemical change in C1. Then, like Dr Jekyll transforming into Mr Hyde, C1 underwent a series of rapid chemical mutations, a 'complement cascade' resulting in the eventual formation of several proteins known collectively as the 'membrane attack complex', or the MAC. The MAC was to a cell membrane what a small stick of dynamite would be to the side of a large brick building. It would put a hole in it.

Most cells could withstand some such punishment, shoring up breaches in their membranes with rapid repairs. But over time, and in sufficient numbers, complement proteins could cause enormous cellular damage. They were a brute-force method for fighting invaders.

McGeer's lab had come up with plenty of evidence that the complement proteins were doing damage in Alzheimer's brains. The proteins were not just in the harmless C1 form. Something was triggering the complement cascade, and C1 was being transformed

---

* Dutch researcher Piet Eikelenboom had reported finding complement in Alzheimer's lesions as early as 1982, though of course no one took notice at the time.
† Complement proteins turn themselves into cell-killing forms through two pathways: the 'classical' and the 'alternative' pathway. The classical pathway is the one that appears principally active in Alzheimer's lesions, and – to avoid too much jargon – is the only one I mean when I refer here to complement activity.

through all its Jekyll-to-Hyde permutations into the membrane attack
complex, which was dynamiting cells left and right.

Naturally, in looking at this evidence, Rogers had searched for
signs that antibodies were present in the lesions of Alzheimer's
brains. Antibodies triggered the complement cascade. And the complement cascade, in these lesions, had been triggered. So antibodies
must have done the triggering.

But though antibodies were quite easy to find, when they were
present, Rogers could not find any – at least no more than the small
background level of them one normally found in the brain. Rogers
admitted this, speaking at the small conference in San Diego, nodding
at the slide images of Alzheimer's brain tissue he had projected on
the screen. He said he was frustrated. He and McGeer had spent
years looking for the cause of all this inflammation in Alzheimer's
brains, and had come up empty-handed.

Outside in the hallway, after his talk, Rogers was having a cigarette
when he was approached by Neil Cooper, an immunologist from the
nearby Scripps Clinic. Cooper had been invited to the meeting as
part of a group of scientists who knew little about Alzheimer's but a
lot about inflammation. Zaven Khachaturian, the meeting organizer,
had been hoping for a cross-pollination of ideas. He got that: Rogers,
you might say, was the flower, and Cooper the bee flying with dust
all over him from the field of immunology.

Cooper mentioned to Rogers that some years before he had found
a few things besides antibody tails that appeared able to bind to
C1 and set off the complement cascade. The list included pieces
of certain obscure parasites and viruses – mainly rat and monkey
RNA leukaemia viruses – and some other small proteins. Cooper
had even published a short paper on it, in 1985, in *Advances in
Immunology*.

Rogers thought that was very interesting: the idea that some
obscure viral protein was triggering the storm of complement. On
the other hand, as he explained to Cooper, he and McGeer had
already searched for viruses in Alzheimer's brains, for an awful long
time, without success.

Rogers flew back to Sun City and pondered the problem. What
could there be, virus or protein, that was triggering the complement
cascade in Alzheimer's lesions? Activated complement proteins were
present in Alzheimer's brains throughout the course of the disease,

from beginning to end. Whatever was setting them off had to be there from beginning to end, too. What was it?

This question was on his mind one day when he stepped up to a microscope in his lab, looked at a stained slice of Alzheimer's brain, and saw the answer staring him in the face.

Beta amyloid.

It was one of those suppositions that suddenly makes a lot of other strange data fall into place. Why did beta amyloid sit at the centre of the disease, yet have no clear-cut direct toxicity to neurons? Because complement was the secret weapon it wielded. Why didn't beta amyloid cause Alzheimer's lesions in mouse models? Perhaps because the mouse complement system wasn't triggered by the human form of beta amyloid the mice were genetically programmed to produce.* Why were all the results on beta amyloid's toxicity to neurons so tricky to reproduce, so weak? Because beta amyloid's toxicity to neurons, if it had any at all, was much less significant than the toxicity of complement.

Since the 1991 Gulf War, television viewers around the world have become familiar with the concept of laser-guided bombing. Over a key target, one plane marks the target with a laser beam, while bombs dropped by other planes home in on the laser spot. It's a simple concept, albeit one that requires advanced computer technology to work properly.

In the body, the same concept had been at work for aeons, with antibodies and complement proteins. The antibody marks the target, and complement proteins zero in and kill it.

Now Rogers believed that beta amyloid, through some random quirk of evolution, had short-circuited the process. It was activating complement all over the place, killing healthy cells. Bombs were dropping where they shouldn't, killing friendly civilians.

Rogers and one of his lab scientists, Scott Webster, started their investigation of this idea with a simple experiment. They took a solution of the protein segment known as C1q, the part of C1 to which an antibody tail bound to activate the cascade. They let the C1q soak into a strip of a paper-like membrane. Then they

---

* At the time of writing, no one has investigated this question.

cooked up various forms of recombinant beta amyloid, along with control proteins, and pipetted drops of them on to the membrane at various points. This was known as a dot blot assay. They rinsed the membrane and sure enough the various lengths of beta amyloid, but not the control proteins, had stuck fast to the Clq.

Showing that beta amyloid stuck to Clq was one thing. Showing that it could set off the complement cascade was another. But there was a relatively simple assay already in use, the CH50 assay, which measured the strength of complement activation. Rogers and Webster added aggregated beta amyloid to the assay. Complement activation began. And the more beta amyloid they added, the hotter the complement activation became. Aggregated beta amyloid bound and activated complement, and seemed to do so about ten times more strongly than Neil Cooper's monkey viruses had done.

Rogers phoned Cooper and suggested that he try similar experiments in his lab. Cooper and his colleague Bonnie Bradt went to it, and using more sophisticated tests they came up with the same results. The same happened up in Vancouver, at Pat McGeer's lab. Eventually a number of other researchers, contacted by Rogers, set about running their own small tests. Even Ivan Lieberburg, the director of research out at Athena Neurosciences, became involved. He and his colleagues showed that beta amyloid bound to Clq so tightly that they could actually use Clq to pull beta amyloid proteins out of solution, a job usually left to highly-specific anti-amyloid monoclonal antibodies.

This was early 1992 and Selkoe and Yankner and others were still arguing over beta amyloid's toxicity or lack thereof. They still had no animal model; the Kawabata–Higgins model had just collapsed. They knew they could engineer mice that accumulated beta amyloid, but they could not find Alzheimer's-type brain damage in those mice.

Rogers now believed, on the strength of the complement experiments, that beta amyloid was indeed a central culprit in Alzheimer's disease, but that it had only a modest direct toxicity to neurons, if any. Its real killing effect, he felt, came when it aggregated into insoluble deposits and, in this form, began to trigger the cell-damaging complement cascade.

Rogers, along with McGeer, saw this amyloid-complement link not just as the key to Alzheimer's – the answer to the long confusion about beta amyloid – but as a possible breakthrough in other areas of immunology. Traditionally, an 'autoimmune disease' was one in which a specific protein in the body was mistakenly targeted by immune cells – immune cells whose receptors were specific for that protein. In multiple sclerosis, for instance, T cells migrated to the brain and targeted the myelin sheaths – the insulators – surrounding nerve axons. Through some unfortunate quirk that combined genetics and circumstances, the immune system's normal checks and balances failed to stop these T cells from going into battle mode. The T cells expanded into a clonal army of anti-myelin beasts that gnawed away on the wires of the brain, destroying connections, killing cells. Something similar happened in diabetes mellitus: because of some genetic flaw in the immune system, plus some unfortunate quirk of circumstance, insulin-producing cells beneath the pancreas somehow came to be seen by the immune system as 'foreign'; an army of T cells grew up and attacked these insulin-producing cells, destroying them all within weeks and removing the body's normal suppliers of insulin.

But with beta amyloid and complement, the 'autoimmune' reaction was different. Neither T cells nor antibodies were involved. Instead a clump of insoluble cellular debris, aggregated beta amyloid, was short-circuiting the complement system, setting off an immunological fire that burned everything in the neighbourhood.

Joe Rogers, along with Pat McGeer, knew that there were many other immunological diseases out there that remained to be explained. Rheumatoid arthritis, for one. Immunologists had long been looking for a T cell clone, or an antibody clone, that caused damage in rheumatoid arthritis. But they had never found one. Rogers believed they might find answers only when they began looking for alternative mechanisms of immunological damage, such as a rogue amyloid-like protein activating the complement cascade.

By now Rogers realized that it was time to start putting his money where his theory was, which is to say he needed to do clinical trials of anti-inflammatory drugs. Other scientists could ignore his retrospective studies, or even the complement work, but direct evidence that patients were being helped by drugs would immediately get everybody's attention.

One of the obvious choices for a drug that should work well

against inflammation in the brain was a corticosteroid known as prednisone. Corticosteroids were chemically related to hormones such as adrenaline that were produced naturally in the human adrenal cortex. They regulated energy burn-rates as well as inflammation. Prednisone, a synthetic version of one of these steroid hormones, was probably the single most powerful anti-inflammatory drug in regular clinical use. It was available in pill form, and, unlike some other drugs, made its way easily from stomach to bloodstream to brain. It was commonly employed to stop the swelling of brain tissue in head injury cases. And it was used to reduce inflammation in severe cases of multiple sclerosis and arthritis.

The prednisone test that Rogers set up was small-scale and informal, and almost cost-free, which was all Rogers could afford. A group of local neurologists, backed by a review board at Boswell Hospital, gave their blessing to the procedure and began to dose four early-stage Alzheimer's patients with prednisone every day. If the patients' dementias had anything to do with chronic brain inflammation, Rogers reasoned, then the prednisone should at least slow the process, and that would be noticeable – so noticeable, thought Rogers, that it would not even be necessary to set up a control group taking placebos. It should be obvious within a few weeks whether there was any change in the patients, and whether a formal, larger-scale, and more expensive trial of prednisone was warranted.

Rogers and his staff briefed the patients' caregivers – nurses, spouses, sons and daughters – and then waited for something to happen. If anything did happen, if any patient suddenly burst out of his demented stupor and became normal again, Rogers wanted to know about it.

When he began taking the prednisone pills, Herbert Sullivan was fifty-eight years old and still living at home in Sun City with his wife, on one of those quiet streets lined with orange and lime trees and yucca plants and well-trimmed grass. Sullivan's Alzheimer's, which Rogers suspected was of the genetic, familial variety, had not progressed very far. Although his memory and personality had decayed, he could still hold a conversation, barely. And he could safely be left alone in the house. His wife worked as an office manager at a local business during the day, leaving Herbert to care for himself at home. She hoped the prednisone would make things even easier for him.

A few days after Herbert had begun taking the drug, his wife did notice some changes. He seemed more energetic. He wasn't really content to sit in his chair any more. Mrs Sullivan had been briefed on the possible side-effects of prednisone. Agitation and restlessness were among those possible side-effects. Prednisone sometimes gave a person more energy than he could safely use. That was another reason Joe Rogers had kept this trial 'open label', without a placebo group. If bad side-effects emerged, he could respond quickly, not having to rummage through his computer to find who was taking the drug. But Mrs Sullivan didn't really see Herbert's energy as a side-effect. She thought Herbert might simply have been emerging, awakening, from his long mental darkness.

One afternoon, while Mrs Sullivan was away at work, Herbert Sullivan got up from his chair and went outside. It was a fine, sunny day. He walked out to the sidewalk, nodded at the neighbours, and continued on down the block. He walked one block, then another block, under the dry blue desert sky. Eventually he came to a grassy embankment that led down to a highway, speed-limit 55. He walked down the embankment. Saw the blue sky up above. The cars whooshing, like multicoloured surf on a blurred grey beach. Also honking. Hollering. Screeching.

Tyres squealed as one car narrowly avoided the man who lurched across the road. Others blared their horns angrily. Somehow Sullivan made it across four lanes without being struck. He walked on to the far shoulder. Found himself amid pebbles, weeds, dirt, shards of glass. And faced another green embankment that ran up, into space, into the sky.

He turned around and walked back out on to the highway.

Joe Rogers, stunned by the news of Sullivan's death, began calling the neurologists and nurses and others involved in the prednisone trial. Stop the trial, he told them. Stop everything.

Rogers would come to believe that prednisone was one of the worst drugs he could have used. At low, safe dosages, he suspected, it would not reach concentrations in the brain sufficient to stop the inflammatory reactions in amyloid plaques. At higher dosages, it appeared, it would cause too much agitation. It would make patients dangerously unmanageable. And that wasn't the only potential problem. There was evidence to suggest that, instead of alleviating dementia, prednisone could make it worse. A group of NIH-sponsored psychiatrists, writing in an issue of the *American Journal of Psychiatry*, had noted strong cognitive impairment – impairment of recall and attention-span – in experimental subjects given some corticosteroids, including prednisone. The steroid's beneficial effects against inflammation, Rogers believed, were outweighed in dementia cases by its dangerous side-effects.

In the fall of 1992, Rogers's paper on beta amyloid and complement appeared in *Proceedings of the National Academy of Sciences*. There was, as usual, no mention of it in the media. American science journalists, watching their fax machines for the latest news from the beta amyloid front, apparently remained unaware that inflammation was even a factor in Alzheimer's disease. But there were ripples of attention among Alzheimer's researchers, not only in academia but in biotech company laboratories, whence Rogers began to receive invitations to come and lecture about his work. He knew that whatever else happened, the inflammation hypothesis was here to stay.

Rogers was now working on his second small-scale clinical trial, this one involving a safer drug, indomethacin. A 'non-steroidal anti-inflammatory drug' (NSAID), indomethacin was related to ibuprofen, and – less closely – to ordinary aspirin. It was most commonly prescribed for arthritis. As Rogers's and McGeer's studies had shown, people who took such drugs for their arthritis were less likely to get Alzheimer's than people who didn't. So NSAIDs seemed like good choices for a basic, first-generation Alzheimer's palliative. They were cheap, they slowed the activities of immune cells, and they were relatively safe for long-term use. Rogers chose indomethacin in particular because it was better than other NSAIDs at getting from the bloodstream into brain tissue, where it would have to get if it was to damp an Alzheimer's inflammatory reaction.

Rogers had grants from the National Institutes of Health and other public agencies, plus funds from philanthropic organizations in Sun City. But these grants were for lab work only, not a clinical trial – and anyway even a moderately-sized clinical trial of a cheap generic drug would cost more than he had in his budget. Setting up protocols and making sure nurses and doctors followed them;

paying neurologists and other specialists for their time; frequently monitoring and testing patients – it all added up quickly. And it was the main reason that, in addition to the normally high cost of producing drugs, pharmaceutical companies had to spend tens if not hundreds of millions of dollars before they brought a new therapy to the FDA.

Of course, no drug company would want to sponsor an indomethacin trial. Indomethacin was an old drug; its main patents had expired years ago. With all the cheap generic versions of indomethacin out there in pharmacies, no company would ever anticipate enough profit to make clinical trial costs worthwhile.

So Rogers had to go it alone, running only a small, exploratory trial. Over several months he enrolled forty-four early-stage Alzheimer's patients around Sun City. Half he randomly assigned to a placebo group, and the other half to the indomethacin group. Patients were not told what group they were in, nor were their doctors or caregivers told. They were simply given a supply of white pills, to be taken thrice daily for six months.

Rogers knew that the size of the trial was almost too small to be useful. The statistical power of comparing two groups of twenty-two patients was very low, especially when the yardstick used to compare the two groups – scores on mental status exams – was somewhat fuzzy anyway. But Rogers felt confident that something would come of it. Some result dramatic enough to make the rest of the Alzheimer's research community pay attention, perhaps bringing in NIH funds for larger and more powerful studies.

Rogers began to work the indomethacin trial, and it wasn't easy. Even with only a few dozen patients to cover, the constant monitoring, phoning, and hand-holding were just about at the limit of what he and his small staff could accomplish. And along the way, patients kept dropping out. Most of the dropouts complained of gastrointestinal problems. Rogers knew they were in the indomethacin group. Indomethacin, like other NSAIDs, tended to irritate the stomach and intestines, especially at high dosages. By the end of six months, there were only fourteen patients left taking indomethacin.

The good news, for Rogers, was that four of the placebo patients had dropped out, too, for another reason: their disease had progressed so rapidly during the six months that they had lost the ability even to sit for a mental status test. Those in the placebo group who hadn't dropped out also had gone downhill, according to the tests.

But that hadn't happened with the indomethacin patients. By and large, their mental scores were the same at the end of six months as they had been at the beginning. And not one of the indomethacin patients had dropped out because of mental deterioration. The indomethacin, rough as it had been on their insides, seemed to have stopped their Alzheimer's disease.

As the news about the indomethacin trial slowly spread, the media at last began to take notice. Rogers and Pat McGeer were the subject of two broadly favourable articles about their work, one in the British magazine *New Scientist*, and another for the research news section of the journal *Science*. The articles described the indomethacin trial and all the suggestive epidemiological evidence that had come before it – the hospital studies, the lepers taking dapsone – as well as the interest the hypothesis was attracting from industry. Ivan Lieberburg, chief scientist at Athena Neurosciences and a key ally of Dennis Selkoe at Harvard, commented in *New Scientist* that 'it's people like Joe Rogers and Pat McGeer who continued to hammer away on this inflammation issue and to say, "Look, this is right under your noses here; this looks like chronic arthritis of the brain – why do you continue to ignore this?"' Even Bruce Yankner, asked by *Science* whether he thought inflammation caused damage in Alzheimer's, admitted, 'I think that has to be considered as a possibility.'

The *New Scientist* and *Science* pieces didn't lead to coverage elsewhere in the media. There was no snowball effect. But the modest amount of attention he and McGeer were getting convinced Rogers that things were looking up. He quickly set about organizing a new trial, this time with 120 patients, some of whom would take dapsone, and some indomethacin. Rogers didn't know how he would manage all those people, with the still-meagre resources at his disposal. But somehow anything seemed possible now.

It was at this point that Mildred Weller came in. Contacted by her husband Max, one of the philanthropists who had helped set up the Sun Health Research Institute, Rogers enrolled Mildred as one of the patients in the new study. There were three groups in the study – placebo, dapsone, and indomethacin – and Max knew fairly quickly that Mildred had been assigned to the indomethacin group, because of the stomach trouble she began to have. The stomach trouble was worse than he had imagined it would be. After a few weeks, it was clear that Mildred, whatever her improvements in mental status, was in agony. She was taken off the drug.

By this time it was also becoming clear to Rogers that the entire trial was beginning to collapse. The indomethacin dosage was higher in this trial than in the first test, and patients were dropping out by the dozens because of the side-effects. Dapsone had a bad side-effect too: haemolytic anaemia, which was more common in Roger's patients than the literature suggested it should have been. The other problem was the scale of the management required to run 120 patients. It seemed like the phone just wouldn't stop ringing.

After two months of near chaos, Rogers decided to fold the trial.

7

The Finish Line

Joe Rogers and Pat McGeer were never really able to taste the victory they had once thought would be theirs. Their years in the wilderness ended, the great day of reckoning came, and went – but without fanfare, and without triumph. The paradigm shifted too smoothly. By the mid 1990s those who studied microglial cells, complement proteins, and proposed testing anti-inflammatory drugs on Alzheimer's patients had little trouble getting attention from serious high-profile journals as well as the popular press. When Duke University researcher John Breitner published a retrospective study of elderly twins, showing that those chronically dosed with anti-inflammatories – especially ibuprofen – had a strikingly low incidence of Alzheimer's, his findings were reported on television and in newspapers around the world. And the idea that beta amyloid deposits could kill neurons, by serving as a constant spark in a spreading immunological fire, became orthodox. Normal. But still hardly anyone outside the Alzheimer's research community had heard about the work of Joe Rogers and Pat McGeer.

In 1995 the National Institutes on Aging decided to take its own look at the McGeer and Rogers strategy with a trial of an anti-inflammatory drug in Alzheimer's patients. On the basis of some preliminary studies by a researcher named Ken Davis, they decided to use prednisone. Joe Rogers wasn't sure what made him angrier: the fact that they were fooling with prednisone, a drug that had already agitated one Alzheimer's patient into the path of a car on a busy freeway, or the fact that the NIA hadn't even bothered to ask his advice. In a stiff, three-page letter to Leon Thal, then heading the NIA's Alzheimer's clinical trials consortium, Rogers noted that 'virtually none of the scientists who opened, developed, and have the greatest knowledge about this area of research were invited to provide input into the consortium's decision. It has been for us a decade's long and very tough battle to get the attention of mainstream scientists such as yourself and the other consortium members. It is even tougher to have you leave us behind at the finish line.'

Rogers continued his lab work, continued to raise money for the Sun Health Research Institute, and continued, with Pat McGeer, to try to organize a new clinical trial of an anti-inflammatory drug. One idea was to use indomethacin again, but also to give patients misoprostol, a drug that alleviated the gastrointestinal symptoms of the NSAID. But Rogers and McGeer couldn't get the money together for a trial large enough to prove anything. Another idea was to try thalidomide, the old horror drug that had deformed hundreds of babies in the 1960s. Thalidomide, then prescribed for morning sickness in pregnant women, also had strong anti-bacterial and anti-inflammatory properties. The FDA would eventually approve it for tests in (non-pregnant) leprosy patients. But the drug regulatory agency turned down Rogers's request for a trial in Alzheimer's patients.

Further distracting from Rogers's and McGeer's achievement was the fact that inflammation wasn't the only new thing being looked at in Alzheimer's research. Perhaps as a delayed effect of all the money pouring into the study of the disease, and all the confusion and anger that had surrounded the issue of beta amyloid's toxicity, Alzheimer's research laboratories suddenly seemed to be going in every direction at once. In fact so many well-funded labs were now contributing to the search for Alzheimer's cause and cure, and were announcing new findings to the press so often, and in such thematic variety, that the newspaper-reading layman could have been excused for thinking that Alzheimer's had become an unsolvable mystery, a chaos where all hypotheses were confirmed but none really worked – where the possibilities somehow never converged.

Even Dennis Selkoe, in a review article for *Science*, would feel compelled to admit, with a hint of lamentation, that 'New research findings on Alzheimer's disease emerge at a furious pace, at first appearing to obscure rather than illuminate a cause of the disease.'

Gone, in other words, was the total dominance of the beta amyloid hypothesis. Even longer gone was the orderly hegemony of the acetylcholine hypothesis – except that a cholinergic drug, tacrine (brand name Cognex) had now been approved by the FDA. This approval was based on large-scale studies in which, the FDA's advisory panel had noted, it had shown a barely noticeable effect. The effect of yelling more loudly at a man almost dead. But with nothing else available, there seemed little reason not to allow such products on to the market. Warner Lambert, the manufacturer of Cognex, was soon pulling in hundreds of millions of dollars from the drug. A similar but less toxic drug made by Pfizer, 'Aricept', reached the market in early 1997.

Around that time a clinical study in the *New England Journal of Medicine* reported weakly positive effects for two anti-oxidant drugs, selegeline and vitamin E. Anti-oxidants work by trapping or otherwise defusing oxygen 'free radicals' before they can fully damage cells and DNA. Oxygen free radicals are by-products, exhaust products, of ordinary metabolic processes in the body, and the damage they cause to cell membranes and DNA – 'oxidative stress' – was by the mid 1990s suspected to be a major cause of ageing in general. Now the notion circulated, in the wake of the *New England Journal* paper, that oxidative stress to brain-cells was also a prime cause of Alzheimer's, and selegeline and vitamin E cheap and simple solutions. But so weak were the effects of the drugs in the study (the combination of selegeline and vitamin E seemed *worse* for patients than either one alone), and so convoluted were the statistical methods used to attain those effects, that the chief of the FDA's drug approval division, Paul Leber, co-wrote an editorial in the *New England Journal* warning in gentle language that the study was virtually worthless.*

There was, by contrast, almost no dispute about the importance of the work pioneered by Allen Roses and his team at Duke University, showing that even late-stage Alzheimer's disease was in some way genetic. Roses's focus was apolipoprotein-E, a protein found in many tissues and involved, among other things, in carrying cholesterol around the body. The gene coding for apo-E was found on chromosome 19 and came in three basic variants – in genespeak, three

---

* Leber co-wrote the editorial with Joe Rogers's old boss from U-Mass, David Drachman.

'alleles' – termed E2, E3, and E4. Because every normal human has two copies of chromosome 19, every normal human has two copies of the apo-E gene, which therefore exist in any of six common allele combinations: E2/E2, E2/E3, E2/E4, E3/E3, E3/E4, and E4/E4.

Allen Roses found, simply, that elderly people who had at least one copy of the E4 allele were several times more likely to have Alzheimer's at any given age than people who didn't. And the E4 allele wasn't rare. In the US Caucasian population, about one out of every four people was E4-positive. The combination of that huge population at risk with the strength of the risk itself helped to explain why Alzheimer's disease was so big. A study published in 1996 by a group of scientists at the University of Washington in Seattle found that elderly people with one copy of E4 had roughly three times the chance of getting Alzheimer's of those who didn't. Those with the E4/E4 genotype, meaning those with two copies of E4, had roughly *thirty* times the chance. Meanwhile there were rare populations, for instance the natives on the Pacific island of Guam, who had almost no E4 in their gene pool – and almost never suffered from Alzheimer's.*

What made these results so intriguing was that for the first time they suggested that late-onset Alzheimer's really did deserve the label of 'disease'. One could have argued, in years past, that the accumulation of beta amyloid deposits in a seventy-year-old Alzheimer's victim merely represented a slight acceleration of the normal, inevitable neurodegeneration of ageing. After all, nearly every seventy-year-old, healthy or not, had some deposits of beta amyloid in his or her brain; it had seemed that there was an age for everyone by which Alzheimer's dementia would set in. But Allen Roses's work on apo-E4 suggested that Alzheimer's wasn't quite so inevitable. Some people would get it, and perhaps some people would not. Perhaps after a certain age the only people still free of Alzheimer's would be those who lacked the E4 allele – an allele that, by the way, was also implicated in atherosclerosis, an unsurprising finding given apo-E's role in transporting cholesterol. One study would find that people who made it to 100 were half

---

* Unfortunately, Guamanians suffered from unusually high rates of other neurodegenerative diseases, including a Parkinsonism/dementia complex that featured a heavy load of neurofibrillary tangles – but no beta amyloid deposits.

as likely to have apo–E4 among their genes as the population as a whole.

The bottom line was that E4 was bad news.

Unfortunately, no one knew what the E4 allele actually did, or didn't do, to increase the risk of Alzheimer's. One series of studies showed that E4 bound more strongly to beta amyloid than did other alleles. A lab at drug giant Eli Lilly & Co., a collaborator of Athena Neurosciences, found that transgenic mice overproducing beta amyloid – who normally accumulated amyloid in clumps in their brain – did not accumulate amyloid when they lacked the gene for apo–E. And mice only have one allele for apo–E: the E4 allele. That suggested that E4 somehow helped beta amyloid to aggregate or accumulate.

Suddenly a lot of laboratories were looking at the cholesterol analogy. Cholesterol problems in arteries, after all, started as loose fatty deposits, then proceeded to clump into hard, brittle, insoluble plaques. Very much like beta amyloid in Alzheimer's brains. And E4 was implicated in both. Alzheimer's researchers – Dennis Selkoe included – began to make friends with atherosclerosis experts.

On the other hand, Pat McGeer's lab found that E4 – but not E3 or E2 – seemed to enhance the ability of beta amyloid to activate complement. Another lab found that E4 interacted with a powerful immune chemical known as interleukin–2. What did it all mean? Sometimes it seemed that laboratory technology was so advanced, nowadays, that it enabled everyone to see what they wanted to see.

And the questions and possibilities continued to blossom outwards. One study found that oestrogen supplements for post-menopausal women reduced the risk of Alzheimer's. Another study, a long-term analysis of a group of nuns, concluded that the ones most resistant to Alzheimer's in later life were those whose writing styles, even at an early age, had a relative richness and complexity – with more of Nabokov, let us say, and less of Hemingway.

In mid 1997 another burst of confusion arrived with a finding by the husband and wife team of John Trojanowski and Virginia Lee at the University of Pennsylvania. In testing some monoclonal antibodies they had grown, antibodies that should have bound to segments of neurofibrillary tangles, Trojanowski and Lee found instead that the antibodies bound to a new protein, 100 amino acids long, that was spread throughout brain areas affected by

Alzheimer's. The new protein seemed more closely associated with dead and dying cells than were NFTs, and seemed to rival beta amyloid as an indicator of the disease, especially because this new protein appeared only rarely in other neurodegenerative diseases. It had been missed, for the ninety years Alzheimer's disease had been around, because pathologists studying the disease had continued to rely primarily on silver and thioflavin to stain tissue. Silver and thioflavin brought out amyloid plaques and NFTs in sharp detail, but didn't enhance the visibility of the new protein and its surrounding plaques. Prominent scientists in the Alzheimer's community, asked for comment by reporters, had to admit that the new protein could become central to Alzheimer's research – which now seemed farther from a conclusion than ever.

To Dennis Selkoe, there was less confusion, and more conclusion, than met the public eye. The new lesion found by Trojanowski and Lee, it turned out, was not really independent of beta amyloid. Beta amyloid was still the key to the disease. It arrived first, when neurons were hale and whole, and it was still there when those neurons were dead and dying. Apo-E4 might be important, but probably through its effects on beta amyloid – possibly by helping it to aggregate in insoluble clumps. Oxidative stress might also be important, but again, it probably worked hand in hand with beta amyloid. Oxygen free radicals were produced, for example, by microglia that had been activated by beta amyloid.

The genetic data, Selkoe saw, had now also converged. The most common types of mutations in early-onset Alzheimer's victims, mutations to genes on chromosomes 1 and 14, had been studied and found to increase the production of beta amyloid, probably through their effects on the enzymes that cut beta amyloid out of its precursor protein, APP. In other words, all the pathways of disease in Alzheimer's apparently led to the build-up of amyloid and, only after that, the deaths of neurons. Neurofibrillary tangles were almost certainly secondary, a result – part of a change in neuron metabolism perhaps – rather than a cause.

It was true that Selkoe now essentially accepted the idea that inflammation played a major role in the disease. 'I am more and more impressed' – he told me in mid 1997 – 'that what Joe Rogers and Pat McGeer have been saying is very sensible.' Selkoe, one of the most cautious, precise speakers I have ever encountered, thus conceded a lot. But he could afford to. He had not lost the Alzheimer's race. Not at all. The race, now, was primarily about developing a drug to eliminate the disease. And Selkoe looked set to win that race.

The drug that would work, Selkoe believed, was one that stopped the build-up of beta amyloid. No beta amyloid meant no toxicity, and no inflammation, and no storm of free radicals, and therefore no disease. Early in the 1990s, on the advice of Selkoe, Ivan Lieberburg's team at Athena Neurosciences in San Francisco had initiated a drug-screening programme. Ironically, given how much sexy, cutting-edge biotech knowhow had been levelled at Alzheimer's, Athena's approach involved a brute-force technique: mass screening of synthetic drug compounds, in the manner of old-fashioned drug companies.

A cell culture had been developed, in Selkoe's lab, that produced recombinant APP and processed some of that APP into beta amyloid, as neurons did. Such amyloid-producing cell cultures were used by Athena and then collaborator, Eli Lilly. The cells hundreds of eight-by-twelve-well plastic laboratory plates. Then the robot arm of a machine pipetted samples of a different drug compound into each of the wells, and another series of devices analysed whether the production of beta amyloid went up or down. The idea was to find a drug that greatly reduced the processing of APP into beta amyloid.

APP was – is – a long protein that normally protrudes from the membrane of a cell. Most of the time, the part of the protein situated outside of the cell eventually encounters an enzyme (dubbed 'alpha secretase') that snips it at a point just above the cell membrane. Imagine one of those razor commercials, where the blade shaves the whisker at an infinitesimal distance from one's chin. That is what alpha secretase does to APP. And as it happens, this cleavage point lies just about in the middle of the beta amyloid section of APP. So most of the time APP is cleaved in such a way that beta amyloid is destroyed.

But a fraction of the time, and perhaps more often when whatever causes Alzheimer's is active, APP never encounters alpha secretase. It hangs there from the membrane of its host neuron, and time goes by, and alpha secretase fails to happen along – and the lonely APP instead is cleaved by another enzyme, 'beta secretase', at a point further out from the membrane – a point at one end of the beta amyloid segment.

The upper part of APP then floats away while the lower fragment, containing beta amyloid, sinks back inside the neuron. And there the remaining cut, freeing beta amyloid, is made by a third enzyme, 'gamma secretase'.* Apparently that is how beta amyloid is produced. Dennis Selkoe believed that the drug that would become the first big Alzheimer's-beater would work by inhibiting one or both of these two enzymes – beta and gamma secretase – that cleaved beta amyloid out of APP.

By 1996, having tested thousands of compounds provided by Eli Lilly, Athena's scientists and technicians had isolated two that strongly inhibited the production of beta amyloid in the special cell cultures. When tested in transgenic mice that overproduced beta amyloid – and normally accumulated insoluble clumps of the stuff throughout their brains – the compounds decreased the formation of the amyloid clumps. Now it is being tested in other animals for side-effects. That has encouraged Lilly to consider applying to the FDA for initial safety trials in humans.

When I visited Selkoe in Boston we sat and talked in his office, small and remarkably undecorated but grandly perched in a brand-new building just off Longwood Avenue. The years had settled lightly on Selkoe, though he now wore bifocals for reading up close. His sandy hair was beginning to turn grey.

But his mind seemed in no way diminished and over a takeout lunch he managed to deliver rapid and detailed and lucid answers to my scattershot questions, his thoughts complete with footnotes, and with all subordinate concepts and clauses and digressions accounted for by the time he finished. Selkoe told me about the two anti-amyloid compounds Athena and Lilly had found. 'They should start testing one of them in people late next year,' he said. In other words late 1999.

If everything goes well, larger-scale trials will start the following year. And, let us hope, a drug to prevent amyloid accumulation – and thus, perhaps, Alzheimer's disease – will become available at pharmacies around 2004.

So in all probability Dennis Selkoe will never get Alzheimer's. Thanks, in large part, to Dennis Selkoe. As we talked, and glaucous

---

* Despite the fact that these enzymes already have names, no one has isolated and sequenced any of them.

summer thunderclouds gathered outside the window, I had the sense
that here was a man about to breeze through a tremendous finish
line, the one he had been focused on since his youth. And here in
his spartan office, in his greying early fifties but with the prospect of
multiple productive decades to come, he would be forced to confront
the question: What next?

When I first met him in person, after several years of telephone
and e-mail and fax correspondence, Pat McGeer was about to turn
seventy years old. He still played tennis every lunchtime, on the
grass court in his backyard. His house lay at the north-west edge
of the University of British Columbia campus, on a tall-banked
peninsula overlooking the mouth of Barrard Inlet and, to the west,
the Strait of Georgia. He had two sons, one daughter, and so far two
grandchildren. He was a professor emeritus. And still he worked
twelve hours a day. And looked, I would say, about fifty-five. A spry
fifty-five.

We sat in his office on a rainy spring afternoon and I asked
him about Alzheimer's. The tangles. The burning plaques. I was
embarrassed to have to ask, but – was he worried about ever
succumbing to the disease himself? Was he taking anything as a
precaution?

He chuckled, said nothing for a moment, but then admitted that
he had indeed been practising what he preached. Every day now,
more or less, he took a dose or two of an anti-inflammatory drug.
Which one? I asked, expecting to recommend it to elderly relatives.
But he wouldn't be drawn on that. 'I don't stick to any one,' he said,
smiling, shrugging. 'I vary them.'

Not long before I first interviewed Rogers for this book, he travelled
north – this was 1996 – for a summer of work alongside Pat and Edie
McGeer in their lab in Vancouver. Rogers, driving up with his wife
and children, phoned the McGeers a day or so ahead of time to say
he would be late. A couple of days later Pat McGeer opened the
Vancouver paper and, there in the sports pages, read why: a golfer
from Arizona, a fellow named Joe Rogers with a Mississippi drawl,
had arrived unexpectedly for a tournament at a course a few dozen
miles outside Vancouver, and had won handily.

Rogers and his family made it to Vancouver a few days later, and moved into a rented house. It was a nice house with a patio at the back, and a rose garden. Rogers was sitting in a chair on the patio one afternoon, sipping a Granville Island Pale Ale and admiring the roses, when the telephone rang. He went in and picked up the phone and listened as the handyman who was house-sitting for him down in Glendale told him what was happening. In fact Rogers could hear with his own ears what was happening. A terrific summer storm had swirled in from – Lord knew where – and had swung down over the high deserts of northern Arizona, aimed at Glendale, aimed at Rogers's very house it seemed, and the thing was just a blitzkrieg of hard rain and punching thunderbolts, and shrieking downbursts and vortices – and the doors upstairs, Joe, have just blown off, and it sounds like the roof is about to go—

Three months later, when I visited Rogers in Sun City, he was still living with his family in a rented house, while repairs continued in the one damaged by the storm.

Rogers was all right. Despite his late start in science, he was still only fifty-two. He looked fine, felt fine. His golf game had actually improved; he had a scratch handicap now, shot a nice, consistent par. And the lab building across from his office was filling, with a new area for studying Parkinson's disease, and another for studying arthritis. He was busy.

And he didn't seem the slightest bit worried about getting Alzheimer's. When I last saw him, on a sunny and warm autumn day in Sun City, he sounded confident that he would never get the disease. His confidence didn't come, however, from the idea of future Alzheimer's treatments, their designs inspired by his work. Instead his reasoning was plain Mississippi fatalism. 'The people in my family tend not to live long enough to get Alzheimer's,' he told me, smoking a cigarette and leaning back reflectively in his office chair. Atherosclerosis of the brain's arteries, he explained, was the family curse instead. 'We tend to stroke out when we're still in our sixties.'

8

The Wall

Stroking out in your sixties. And now in your early fifties. A shorter wait, in other words, than many murderers now on death row. But at least there would not be the torture of Alzheimer's.

If you want to become a little depressed, sit quietly for a minute and try to fit your mind around Alzheimer's disease: the millions of patients, gray, unfocused, the humanity draining from them daily in homes and hospitals and nursing facilities around the world. Mildred Weller with her headphones on, hearing but not really listening to Glenn Miller. In the Mood.

In the United States those with Alzheimer's comprise about 1.4 per cent of the population, one out of seventy people. If you add those whose plaques and tangles are silently accumulating and will go critical within a few years, the figure probably rises to around one in fifty people. And that neurological holocaust is only one side of the disease. On the other side are the scientists, with their herd-like movements down dead-end trails, their rivalries, ambitions, wandering prophecies, rises and falls. I have told the story, a story, of Alzheimer's research from one narrow perspective, and as any scientist I've failed to mention will tell you, I've barely scratched the surface. Yet I find even this small part of the story exhausting. All that energy; all those concentrated minds and lives. And, really, so little accomplished. By a species that already has sent its men to the Moon, its ships billions of miles into interstellar space.

And here is the most depressing fact of all: if Alzheimer's research were to succeed tomorrow – if the disease suddenly went the way of smallpox and the plague – the average lifespan of humans would increase by . . . perhaps two years, perhaps less. Another couple of dozen rounds of golf. Another few seasons in the sun. Because at that

age there are so many other things that can kill you. You will stroke
out. Or drop from a heart attack. Or get the cancer. Remember, Man,
that you are dust.

Of course there are other, even larger societies of scientists and
patients suffering and straining to defeat those other big killers.
There are many other stories.

Strokes and cardiovascular illness are both part of the same story
because they are different results of the same general disease: vascular
disease, the thickening and hardening and eventual blockage or
rupture of blood vessels. In a heart attack a coronary artery is
blocked, and part of the heart muscle dies. In strokes an artery feeding
the brain is blocked, and part of the brain dies. Atherosclerosis, the
term for the process that comprises most vascular disease, begins
with fatty streaks inside artery walls, these streaks being made up
largely of macrophages, garbage-gobbling immune cells, that have
gorged themselves on fat molecules. The fatty streak gradually sinks
into the arterial wall and becomes a thick, brittle plaque, full of fatty
stuff, and overgrowing smooth-muscle cells, and fibrous material of
the kind produced by the body to close wounds.

Somehow cholesterol-based molecules known as LDL, low-
density lipoprotein, push this process along. Molecules known as
HDL, high-density lipoprotein, slow it down. Sitting around and
watching TV, and eating potato chips, and getting old, tends to
lower HDL levels and increase LDL levels. Getting exercise and
eating a low-fat diet, and taking anti-cholesterol drugs – and having
lots of oestrogen in your body, as you do if you're a pre-menopausal
woman – has the opposite effect.

Anti-cholesterol drugs do their business in various ways, but
one popular class – which includes Upjohn's Colestid – binds to
bile acid, an intermediate link in the body's cholesterol-processing
chain, and effectively flushes it out. One more promising contender
is GelTex Pharmaceuticals' CholestaGel, now in clinical trials in the
US. Essentially a plastic molecule that binds to bile acid, GelTex
does what other bile-binding drugs do, but with few or none of
their gastrointestinal side effects. More ambitious strategies include
gene therapies to super-charge the liver so it processes LDL out
of the bloodstream more efficiently, and drugs that whittle down
existing LDL-based plaques. On the dietary side, there are efforts

to invent various fat substitutes that pass through the body without ever collecting in arteries, while other scientists – at Amgen Co., for instance – are busy developing biotech drugs, bred from human genes, that will simply make obese people feel less hungry, and eat less fat.

Vascular disease is number one on the list of killers in the developed world. Number two on the list is cancer, a fundamental disease of organisms: an uncontrolled proliferation of cells. Death from cancer is, in a sense, death from too much life.

There are many cancers, and that is so because there are many ways a cell can be made to grow cancerously. There are many ways its genes can be deranged. There are genes that when mutated do something they should not, such as push a cell towards uncontrolled division. There are genes that when mutated fail to do something they should, such as suppress uncontrolled growth. Cancerous cells are not really human cells any more; they are little monsters, their once-orderly chromosomes, designed to work in harmony with their cellular neighbours, now like ruthlessly selfish, ever-mutating viruses. But they are human enough that they present a more challenging target to the immune system than a virus–infected cell. And unlike a virus, which might have only a few dozen genes at its disposal, a cancerous cell has the entire human genome from which to choose its deadly proliferative strategies.

Still, there are reasons to think that cancer will become steadily less of a threat, at least for people who are not extremely old. For one thing, the cure rates for most cancers already have been rising dramatically over the past few decades, thanks to new techniques such as bone-marrow transplants, and more efficient chemotherapy drugs. Those new techniques and chemo drugs will probably soon be outdated by some novel treatments on the horizon.

One of the most interesting anti–cancer strategies now being looked at doesn't even go after tumours directly. Instead it attacks the blood vessels on which tumours depend.

When a cell turns cancerous in the body it gives birth, by repeatedly doubling and doubling, to a clonal clump of cancerous cells. When this clump of cells gets to a diameter of about a sixteenth of an inch – a harmless size, generally speaking – it reaches a threshold. To grow larger, it must have blood. And to have blood, it must persuade nearby blood-vessels to sprout new tendrils, to connect it to the body's main energy grid. Tumours that do this, and make it past the blood supply threshold, usually do so by pumping out a lot of blood-vessel growth factors – causing blood-vessels to grow into and around it just as explosively as the tumour itself is growing.

Back in the 1980s, Professor Judah Folkman of Boston's Children's Hospital and the Harvard Medical School decided that this explosive blood-vessel growth would make a good target for an anti-cancer therapy. The vessels themselves are not cancerous; they can't mutate around drugs the way tumour cells do. After years of sifting through various compounds, Folkman's lab came up with two promising ones, dubbed angiostatin and endostatin, both of them fragments of naturally occurring proteins. Used in combination, in mice, they worked very well: they seemed to cure such a range of cancers that the *New York Times* put them on its front page in early May 1998 and caused a full-blown media bubble – which only subsided when reporters discovered that scientists have been curing cancer in mice for years, and that humans, alas, are much harder to treat successfully. Angiostatin and endostatin haven't been tested yet in humans; though they should be soon, in a clinical trial sponsored by the National Cancer Institute. That trial is currently being held up by the difficulties Bristol-Myers-Squibb, the drugs' licensee, has had in mass-producing a big protein like angiostatin.

Similar difficulties have sidelined a lot of other 'angiogenesis-inhibitor' drugs, although twenty so far have made it into clinical trials, and a second generation of drugs is on the way. One of these second-generation drugs, developed at the Burnham Institute in La Jolla, California, is an easy-to-make peptide that zeroes-in on receptors found only on tumour-supplying blood-vessel cells. The peptides carry the chemo drug doxorubicin to the cells, and kill them, thereby quickly starving the tumours. That happens in mice, anyway; clinical trials in humans should start in 1999.

Other anti-cancer strategies include: cancer vaccines that target antigens found only on cancer cells; monoclonal antibodies that block the activity of mutant cancer-promoting proteins; and viruses and proteins that can infiltrate cancer cells and throw a biological self-destruct switch, causing the cells to commit suicide.

The much-hyped 'gene therapy' will probably also be brought

to bear. In one approach, developed by gene therapy pioneers Michael Blaese and Kenneth Culver at NIH, a tumour is first injected with cells that produce a special gene-carrying virus, a 'vector' in genespeak. This vector spreads from the injected cells and infects some of the nearby cancer cells, delivering into them a special gene. This gene codes for a special enzyme, thymidine kinase (tk). Thymidine kinase can convert the antiviral drug gancyclovir into a compound that shuts down DNA synthesis, and thereby effectively kills any cancerous cell in which it is active. So with this enzyme in place in some of the cancerous cells, the patient is given a dose of gancyclovir – and the tk-carrying cancer cells, and all neighbouring cancer cells within reach of the seeping DNA-shutoff-compound, are snuffed out. Results in mice have been outstanding, and though early results in humans have been, as usual, less dramatic, the tk/gancyclovir approach clearly represents a good start. In any case, with all these new drugs becoming available – and I imagine them being used in combinations, in 'cocktails', like the current Aids drugs – I can't help thinking that twenty or thirty years from now most cancers will be as treatable as bacterial diseases are today.

But remember, Man, that you are dust. If science could remove, tomorrow, not just Alzheimer's disease but also vascular disease and cancer from the arsenal of death, the Grim One would still have plenty of other weapons to choose from. Diabetes, kidney failure, liver failure, or immune system failure that leaves you defenceless against infections. You, however vigorous and healthy at threescore and ten – no more cancer! no more Alzheimer's and atherosclerosis! – would still be lucky to make it to fourscore and ten. The expected lifespan, at birth, for an average American or European is now about seventy-five. If we suddenly wiped out Alzheimer's and vascular disease and cancer – and think of the enormity of the effort required to do that; like twenty Manhattan Projects – the average lifespan would move only to about eighty-five. Hardly a quantum, Methuselan leap. We would merely linger a while more in the late autumn of our lives. Playing golf, but driving that ball shorter and shorter distances down the fairway. Playing bridge at the rest home a while longer. Gaping at the droning faces of CNN a while longer. Watching the increasingly blurred shapes of life pass by, a while longer.

Being old a while longer.

Because you are dust. You are what evolution has made you. You are not designed to live for ever. You are, in a sense, designed not to.

How could Evolution have done this to us? Why has our immortal God made us mortal?

To get a sense of the reasons, start by thinking of ageing as a genetic disease, a horrible and fatal disease that suddenly causes your cells to decay when you reach a certain age.

Now, if this genetic disease struck and killed you when you reached the age of eleven, then it would be selected out of the gene pool very quickly. A person who had the gene for this disease* would die before his or her procreative years, and thus would not pass the gene on to the next generation. The gene would disappear.

But let us move the age of onset of this strange disease – this disease called 'ageing', caused by this bad gene – to twenty. Then it becomes possible for the gene to be passed on, because people will have started to breed before then. Of course, the evolutionary pressure will still be against the gene, because the age of twenty is still quite early in the child-producing years. The gene will not be passed on to the next generation as prolifically as other genes, because the gene curtails its own proliferation, by killing its proliferator – you – before it can produce as many copies of the gene as possible.

This evolutionary pressure drops off, however, as the age-of-onset of this disease gets higher, and passes out of the breeding years, and out of the parenting years, and into the grandparenting years. And when the gene doesn't kick in until seventy – even the grandchildren have grown up now, and can fend for themselves – there might even be evolutionary pressure from the other direction. In other words, it might be better, from the perspective of this gene, that you – old duffer – get out of the way and leave more resources for the latest copies of the gene you have already produced.†

*   *   *

* For simplicity I assume here that the ageing gene is dominant, meaning that only one copy, inherited from either mother or father, will be enough to kill you.
† Such a pressure probably didn't exist in the human past, because humans' environment was too harsh to permit them to live that long.

Lord, how cruel that sounds. And from the point of view of human individuals, sentient bodies, it certainly is cruel. Evolution has tended to treat us sentient bodies more or less like disposable machines: machines that protect genes and make copies of them, and then are discarded once they have done so.

But now look at it another way: you can design an organism to resist ageing for a very long time. You – God, Evolution – can build in comprehensive sets of enzymes and proteins and growth factors that repair DNA and strip out unwanted extracellular gunk (cholesterol, amyloid) and keep cells healthy and kicking for centuries. But what is the point of all that effort – surely a huge diversion of bodily resources – when your environment is not going to let you live nearly that long? What if life is always going to be nasty, brutish, and short?

The gangs of genes that roam your chromosomes appear to have learned over a billion years or so that the best way to keep copies of themselves in existence is not by surrounding themselves with some super organism and trying to keep it alive for ever (impossible, in the face of marauding viruses and bacteria and velociraptors and T. Rex) but by crafting one temporary organism, using that to spread copies of themselves, and living on through the copies.

And in all this of course the disposable bodies, those fancy copying machines, are left more or less to languish and decay once they make their copies. Because, again, it is a much better strategy for the gangs of genes – in a harsh world where death is never far away – to put their biological resources into early procreation, massive copying and dissemination, rather than eternal corporeal life. Sex, instead of the avoidance of death. Sex, one of our consolation prizes for being mortal. Sex, to get those genes up to the next generation before T. Rex stomps by.

And that is the simple logic of mortality. Some organisms, some species, have been designed to live only for days. Their environment is that harsh. We humans, by comparison, don't have such a bad deal. We have the luxury, now after all those aeons thinking and fighting our way out of the hot forests and savannas, of taking around thirteen years to reach breeding condition. Thirteen years: already a ripe old age for many large mammals such as dogs and cats. Generally speaking, in higher animals – and there are exceptions, like Pacific salmon – the longer it takes to reach sexual maturity, the slower the subsequent process of ageing. Humans, as Earth species go, take an awful long time to die.

Yet they do die. They fade and grey, and no matter how much exercise they get, no matter what elixirs and creams and potions they take, they hit a biological wall some time around the age of seventy. The great majority of people in developed countries now die before they reach eighty. About one half of 1 per cent totter to ninety. A fiftieth of 1 per cent are wheeled forward to 100, blinking at all those candles. A thin fraction of these drift a bit further, inert now, already embalmed by weird flukes of their genetics, their minds like old fluorescent tubes that buzz and flicker once or twice a day. Do not believe those stories about pockets of 160-year-olds living and dancing in Shangri-La valleys in Mongolia or Uruguay, where the water and air are preternaturally pure. Those are places, simply, where accurate birth records are not kept. A psychology PhD thesis needs to be written about the tendency of some people, once they become wrinkled and grey and stooped, to stop shaving years off their actual age and start adding years on, shovelling and piling them on, up to absurd Methuselan heights.

A few days ago, a few days before writing this, I visited my dentist. It was my first visit in a couple of years. Time for a cleaning. My teeth were actually fairly healthy but I had begun to have the bad dreams about them. Maybe you know what I am talking about. The dreams where you look in the mirror and the molars, canines, incisors, bicuspids are all black and cracked and rotted and falling out. Because you are getting old. And when you wake up, you go to that same mirror, to check – Yes, thank God, still there, uncracked, unrotted.

Things change, in the town where I grew up, but one thing never does. My dentist, Dr O'Brien, always asks me about my cousin Jennifer.

'How is your cousin Jennifer?' he asked me this time, as I spat out the silver fragments of an aged filling he had just replaced.

'Jennifer?' I said. 'Haven't seen her in a while. I think she's living in Connecticut now. Married to a banker' – I am changing some of the personal details here – 'You used to date her, didn't you, Doc?'

He smiled shyly, perhaps ruefully. 'Well, yeah. We had, sort of – a summer of love I guess you could say.'

A summer of love. And now, in his early forties, married, nice house, kids, still trim and athletic-looking but his hair going salt-and-pepper grey. And thinking back. Ah, youth.

When I told Dr O'Brien I was writing a book on ageing he said with a certain fervour, 'I think the key is to enjoy life. See the world. Take time to smell the roses. And find something you like to do. Find a job you really love.'

I wanted to protest – no! I don't want just to live well, I want to live long, for ever! – but he had one of those sharp little tools in my mouth, picking at my teeth, and the sounds I made weren't intelligible.

'You like being a dentist, don't you, Dr O'Brien?' asked his hygienist.

'Well . . . yeah,' he sighed, meaning: maybe not any more.

She laughed. 'Maybe you should play more golf.'

Maybe, instead of accepting ageing and death, people will decide not to. I don't know how this change in consciousness will come about. Already it seems to have started but I don't know if it will continue to proceed slowly or will instead reach a critical point and then just finish suddenly, *whoompf*, like an avalanche, or like everybody hooking up to the Internet a couple of years ago.

But when it finally happens I think we will look around, as if waking from a stupor, and ask ourselves: why are we spending so many billions of dollars to fight age-related diseases when the payoff, in extra years of life, is so slight? Why don't we put more of our resources, many more, into bolder strategies? We don't just want not to die – we want not to be old, stooped, slowed, impotent, prone to falls, intellectually closed. We want youth. We want the rising sap. We want cells with low mileage. We want arteries and brains and limbs unclotted by the gradual detritus of death. High priests of Science! If you are good for anything – give us this!

PHASE TWO
SPARE PARTS

9

The Ordeal of Near-Death

You could play the what-if game. You could ask: what if, in the spring of 1971, the Draft Board of Contra Costa County California had given a seventeen-year-old boy named Carl June a higher draft number?

If they had given Carl June a higher draft number, high enough to keep him out of the draft that year, he would have gone to Stanford University the following September. Carl lived in Contra Costa County, in the town of Pleasant Hill east of Oakland. His father was a chemical engineer. His uncle and grandfather were engineers. Carl would have studied engineering, and maybe played some football. He was a solid-looking kid, six two, two hundred five pounds. He hit you, you felt it. The United States Naval Academy, out east in Annapolis, Maryland, had actually tried to recruit him, had wanted him as an offensive lineman. But Carl had his heart set on Stanford, which already had accepted him into its 1971 freshman class.

Then Carl June got the letter from the Draft Board, notifying him of their recent lottery. Perhaps they had one of those machines in which a fan blows ping-pong balls up in the air inside a clear plastic box, and the balls all have numbers stencilled on them, and a plump girl in a bikini and a smile and a great big '71-model hairdo hits a lever and one of the numbered balls pops up into a little cage. To Vietnam or not to Vietnam.

Carl June's number was fifty, which meant: to Vietnam.

And Stanford was out. And the Naval Academy started to sound a lot better. Hell, if he was going to go to war, he might as well do it as an officer.

June found that he liked the Naval Academy. He didn't stay on the football team; it turned out he wasn't bulky enough. Instead he slimmed down and joined the crew team, and stroked up and down the Severn River through autumn mists, past the drones of wood boats running crab lines near the brackish shores, the verdant cliffs. Already it was clear that the war in Vietnam was ending, for Americans at least. An eighteen-year-old could think about being young again.

After a summer on a destroyer at sea, in monsoonal South East Asia but out of range of the war, the only rumbles those from thunder, June came back to Annapolis and heard about a special programme for Academy students: each year a small number of applicants would be selected for medical training. They would spend the rest of their Academy years doing pre-med work, then would go on to a civilian medical school. All of it would be paid for by the Navy. The only hitch was that the years of obligation to the Navy would really pile up. Five years of obligation for going through the Academy, and another four for medical school, and another three for internship and residency. It was essentially a career decision. By the time June finished serving out all that Navy time, he'd already have put in almost twenty years, so he might as well stay for the full twenty and get the pension.

June was nineteen years old when he made that decision. He was at another what-if point, another fork to an alternate future. In this future he decided to be a doctor. He applied and was accepted to the medical programme, as one of eight in an Academy class of 1100. And three years later he started at Baylor Med School down in Houston. He soon discovered that he loved medicine.

Later he would marvel that he had taken such a path in life. But the truth was that as a teenager back in Pleasant Hill he and his friend Doug Hiteshew had done some impromptu transplant experiments on rats. This had not been biology lab stuff. This had not been homework. This had been a couple of boys devising animal surgery on their own. They had gone into a pet store and bought the rats, and then had anaesthetized them with tetrachloroethylene and cut them open and poked around, and then had sewn them up again – just to see if they could do it.

June finished Baylor in three years, working on an accelerated programme, then went to Geneva for postdoctoral work with the World Health Organization, then did his internship and residency at Bethesda Naval Hospital in Maryland. In 1983 he went to Seattle, to take a postdoctoral fellowship at the Fred Hutchinson Cancer Research Center. The Navy wanted to start up a bone-marrow transplant programme, and was sending a few of its best young physicians for training.

The Hutchinson Center – 'Hutch' – was doing most of the bone-marrow transplant operations in the world then. BMTs were still only experimental. They were dangerous; they were harrowing. When you received a BMT, it was usually because you were close to death from cancer. The doctors at Hutch started by taking you even closer to death, to the howling brink of that abyss – and then they tried to bring you back again.

Carl June was married now, thirty years old, with two young sons aged one and three. The Navy had put him and his family in a gorgeous big Victorian house on a sprawling facility, Magnolia Hill, once an old embarkation point – a muddy hump of tents and quonset huts – in the war against Japan. Looking grandly out over Puget Sound, it was the Seattle version of San Francisco's Presidio. June's house would normally have been given to an admiral, or at least a captain, but it was given to him, Lieutenant June, MD, because it was the only one empty when he arrived. It was a good place to come back to in the evenings, because in town at Hutch he saw death every day, death in its most monstrous and inexorable forms.

One day Carl June was presented with the case of Maria Morderas, a thirty-seven-year-old wife and mother. Maria Morderas had chronic myelocytic leukaemia. White blood cells in her bone marrow – mainly cells known as granulocytes – had gone cancerous and had begun to multiply pathologically, snuffing out the production of oxygen-carrying red blood cells in her marrow and causing anaemia, among other things. Chronic myelocytic leukaemia, left to its own devices, was one hundred per cent fatal, though it took its time about it, coming and going like some awful version of malaria. With supportive medical treatment for her periodic anaemias, Maria could expect to live for another several years before the leukaemia cells mutated into a super-aggressive form and killed her. With a bone-marrow transplant, she had a chance of surviving longer than that, perhaps even living another few decades, cancer-free. Was the chance of that 30 per cent? 40 per cent? Certainly there was a good chance, at least 25 per cent, that she would die much more quickly, perhaps within a few weeks, from complications related to the transplant operation itself. It could go either way. That was one reason the technique was considered experimental.

Another hard thing about the Morderas case was this: Maria's husband had told her only that she was ill with a blood disease. He had not told her that she had cancer. He had not told her that she was probably going to die. It was left to young Doctor June to tell her this.

When Maria Morderas decided to undergo the bone-marrow transplant operation, June and his colleagues began by taking blood samples from her family members, checking the immune markers on their blood cells for matches to her own. The better the match, the better the chances that the operation would succeed.

As luck would have it, they found a perfect match – according to the screening tools of the time – in Maria's brother Carlos. He was not her twin, but immunologically he seemed just about identical. The consent forms were signed, and Maria Morderas's ordeal began.

This ordeal, though still experimental, had already been finely tuned by the doctors at Hutch. It was designed to bring a patient's body to a near-death state – killing it, almost, in order to save it, as some had said of Vietnam.

It all began on day eight pre-op, in other words eight days before the actual transplant. On this day Maria Morderas, wearing a paper hospital gown, was led into a windowless chamber that might well have been called the chamber of near-death. Certainly it could have functioned as a chamber of full death, just as efficiently as, say, a gas chamber or an electric chair facility at a prison. The walls were lined with concrete and lead. Maria was asked, by a white uniformed hospital technician, to lie in a certain position on a low sheet-covered platform. Then the hospital technician left, and closed the heavy door behind her. Maria was alone in the room with a large grey machine, its boxy proboscis hanging over her. It looked like an X-ray machine but in fact it was simpler than that. It merely contained a silvery, molten lump of extremely radioactive caesium, and was designed to expose the caesium, for a closely controlled time, to whomever lay on the platform.

Maria would have heard the click as the shutter opened but would not have felt the horrendous shower of gamma rays tearing through her body. Gamma rays did not give one a definite feeling of warmth upon the skin, as ultraviolet did – you know, that subtle tingling on a cloudy summer day at the beach. The gamma rays had more energy than ultraviolet and they were not stopped by skin; they penetrated more deeply into the body, careening electrons from their orbits, causing chemical changes, creating monster oxidizers, mutators and breakers and fusers that made DNA unrecognizable, unprocessable. Imagine a thin scatter of tiny buckshot fired through the pages of a book, taking out a letter here, half a word there, creating new spellings, new meanings, or confusions that negated the meanings of entire chapters.

Though the heat produced by all these richocheting electrons and chemicals was dissipated imperceptibly throughout her body, Maria probably felt the beginnings of something bad by the time a few minutes of exposure passed and the shutter clicked shut and stopped the caesium shower. There was some kind of receptor system in the brain – God knew how it had evolved – that was sensitive to widespread cellular insults like this. It made Maria Morderas want to throw up.

They say that a charging grizzly bear, shot through the heart, can still cover twenty yards and crush your skull with a great clawed swipe before it knows it has been killed. Its heart beats that slowly. Its powerful grizzly bear system has several seconds of circulating blood and oxygen, several seconds of bear power after every heartbeat, even if that beat is the last.

The situation is similar with a cell in the body, when its DNA has been holed or mutated at many points. It does not die right away. Some of the proteins it tries to manufacture from its genes will not come out right, of course, but perhaps all the important ones will. Only when the cell tries to divide – like that next pump of the grizzly bear heart – will the damage become evident. The little mutations here and there, the occasional obdurate fusings of the nucleotides across the helix, will add up to fatal kinks and breaks in the unfolding DNA. Instead of two new live and growing cells there will be just dead protoplasm, cell stuff, an aborted monster.

Populations of fast-dividing cells, like white blood cells – especially cancerous ones – are therefore the first to die following such a large insult to a body's DNA. Moderately-dividing cells, like hair cells, die a bit later; that is why chemo and radiation therapy patients go bald. Non-dividing cells, such as neurons and heart muscle cells, die hardly at all.

There is a thin threshold here between death and mere near-death. After a certain radiation dose, a certain number of rads per kilogram of body mass, a human being cannot survive unaided for more than a few weeks. The damage goes beyond the body's capacity for endurance and repair.* Below that threshold, however, the body can carry on, can renew itself.

The doctors at Hutch, waiting with their arms folded outside the lead-lined door of the chamber, gave BMT patients doses of radiation that went beyond the threshold. They were 'super-lethal' doses, that is, more than lethal, more than enough to kill you. The radiation did not kill all cells, not by a long shot, but it did completely destroy the most sensitive population of cells: bone-marrow cells. That was good, because the marrow cells were where the cancer was. But that was also bad, because a person needed marrow cells to have blood, to have an immune system.

That was where the marrow transplant came in. When the body had been brought to the brink, the marrow destroyed, new marrow was added from a donor, and the new marrow multiplied and formed a new and healthy system of blood cells in the body. Without such a transplant the patient would die. With the transplant, a 'lethal' dose of radiation could be overcome.

Maria Morderas came out of the chamber of near-death, that first day, and vomited with radiation sickness. Her stomach continued to heave that afternoon, and that night. And the next morning she went into the chamber again, for her second dose.

The prescribed course was six doses in the chamber, over six days, and after each dose Maria went back to her new room in the isolation ward. She lay in a sterilized bed, in a sterilized room. Doctors who

---

* During the Cold War the Pentagon's nuclear war planners calculated that a battlefield nuclear exchange would leave many soldiers with a lethal dose of radiation but without any symptoms other than telltale nausea. Such 'walking ghosts' were naturally a concern. What would they do, knowing they were certain to die in a few days?

entered had to wear surgical gowns and masks and gloves as if they were about to perform surgery in the operating room.

Maria was now being fed through an IV catheter. She could not digest food in the normal way. Her mouth and throat were becoming red, and very, very tender. Epithelial cells, relatively fast dividers, lined the gastrointestinal tract. Their deaths – and they were dying now by the billions – were turning this tract, from lips to throat to stomach to intestines and out to the anus, into one long cold sore, a swollen and red stretch of pain. Maria thought it was very bad, but her ordeal had just started. The pain would get much worse, requiring huge doses of morphine. Her moderate hair loss would progress to complete baldness. And there was chemotherapy now. Her marrow cells were probably dead, but just to make sure, the doctors were giving her a super-lethal dose of a chemo drug that did essentially the same thing that radiation did, killing cells that tried to divide. A catheter took her urine and, going the other way, kept her irrigated with water; without this the chemo drug as it exited her body would strip the lining from her bladder and urethra. The lining of her GI tract, meanwhile, was beyond help; it was being sloughed off in the form of frequent, greenish, red-flecked diarrhoea. Maria received daily transfusions of red blood cells and clotting factors. There were IVs of glucose, and medicines and antibiotics. And a constant drip of morphine for the pain. She seldom had visitors, for to see her, up close, her family members had to don the same surgical gowns and masks that doctors and nurses wore. Having no immune system, Maria was defenceless against microbes. She was dizzy, constantly nauseous. She had reached the brink.

Two days after the last dose of radiation Carl June and a colleague and some nurses and assistants took Maria's brother Carlos to an operating room, laid him face down on a table, and gave him epidural anaesthesia. When the man was sufficiently dosed, June and the other doctor each grasped a long, thin, hollow spike of stainless steel, holding it by a special grip – like a corkscrew grip – and twisted it into the back of Carlos's pelvis, above the hip, into the large pelvic bone, the ilium bone. Mining for marrow. When June had penetrated the outer bone and the point of the hollow spike was inside the marrow, he removed the grip from the spike, attached a large syringe instead, and sucked out a thin, dark stream of marrow.

It looked like mushy blood with white bits of bone. The red mush was filtered and collected in a clear plastic marrow bag. When he had sucked out what he could, turning the hollow spike this way and that, June put the grip on again and punched another hole. In this way the two doctors, their hands getting sore and blistered with the effect, worked two or three hundred holes each in Carlos's ilium, from one hip to another around the back, and collected about a quarter-pound of the marrow stuff, enough to fill, by way of illustration, the small cupped hands of Maria Morderas.

June brought the bag of marrow up to the isolation ward, put on new scrubs, and, assisted by a nurse, stuck a catheter into one of Maria Morderas's major veins, just below her neck. The bag of marrow was hung above the bed, a tube was hooked from it to the catheter, and within half an hour all the marrow had drained into Maria's blood. That was all that was necessary, surgery-wise. The marrow cells had molecules on them that naturally and magically homed in on bone. They didn't clog up Maria's blood, didn't give her a heart attack or a stroke. They found their own way into her marrow. They were the seeds of her new blood-supply, her new immune system.

So far, so good, but now came a terrible wait. The greatest single risk in this entire procedure was not death by radiation. As horrible as the chamber of near-death might have seemed, and indeed was, radiologists knew quite well how much radiation the body could stand in the short term. They knew it almost as well as chemists at Kodak knew how much light would overexpose a piece of photographic film. No, the greatest risk here was death from T cells, the very cells that the bone-marrow transplant was designed to restore.

Hopefully, when Carlos's marrow cells seeded themselves within his sister's bones and got comfortable, they would begin to pump out the normal range of blood cells: granulocytes, monocytes, reticulo-cytes, erythrocytes, macrophages, B cells, T cells, and so on. Maria Morderas would have an immune system again, and it would be healthy, all the cancerous cells having died in the nuclear holocaust in the near-death chamber.

Hopefully. But in reality, where hopes didn't always come true, the experimental BMT surgeons at Hutch had been finding that in 25 per cent of cases – and these were cases in which the tissue seemed immunologically matched – the T cells coming out of the newly-seeded marrow were in fact not properly matched: the T cells perceived the surrounding cells of this new body not as 'self' but as 'foreign'. As something to be attacked and killed. They came out of the marrow into the blood, and went into battle mode, and began to proliferate, and attacked cells, holing them with lethal chemicals, gobbling them to death. And soon enough they succeeded in their mistaken mission. They killed the body that housed them. This process was called GVHD: graft versus host disease. When it took hold, in a bone-marrow transplant patient, it often meant that the end was near.

One of the new weapons being used against GVHD at the Hutchinson Center was a drug called 'Sandimmune', better known to scientists and surgeons as cyclosporine. The drug was manufactured by Sandoz, a large Swiss drug company with a plant in New Jersey. Sandoz was running a three-page ad in all the transplant surgery and immunology journals, telling everyone about cyclosporine. The first page had a nifty, abstract, geometric image evoking the cyclic chemical structure of the compound: a formation of stick-figure skydivers, their stick-figure hands linked, and all of them plunging through starry deep space.

Somehow – nobody knew exactly how – cyclosporine interfered with the basic workings of T cells. In the test tube, it kept T cells from becoming activated when they were presented with foreign antigens. T cells, it was thought in those days, were something like fighting cocks. Just give them a taste of the enemy – as cockers always did before a bout – and they would go into battle mode, pumping out chemicals to rally other T cells, and multiplying their numbers, clonally, to form massive armies of enemy-skewering, enemy-gobbling cells. And each T-cell clone (or set of genetically identical cells) had a different shape of antigen receptor – the 'T-cell receptor', or TCR, this was called – that locked on to a specific piece of a foreign antigen, be it a piece of virus, bacterium, parasite, or a cell from somebody else's liver. There were billions of T-cell clones in the body, each specific for a particular protein shape out there in nature. When one of those shapes was encountered by a T cell specific for that protein shape, the T cell 'activated' and began making copies of itself, and the killing started.

Sandoz's drug chemists had found that when they added

cyclosporine to their standard test-tube assays of T-cell activation (usually T cells in a culture medium, with some powerful T-cell-aggravating antigen included) T-cell activation was blocked. And this made cyclosporine a potentially very valuable drug. Control T cells and, medically speaking, you could just about control the world. T cells were the keys to numerous diseases and conditions and problems, and transplant rejection was one of the most important. Stopping transplant rejection – GVHD was one form of rejection, albeit a reversal of the usual host–versus–graft attack – meant stopping T-cell activation. Cyclosporine did that. Not only in the test tube but in mice, and later, almost as well, in clinical trials with humans.

Transplant surgeons already had some drugs they could use to fight transplant rejection. They had methotrexate, a cancer-chemo drug that effectively killed most cells. And they had the old steroid standby, prednisone, which killed T cells and suppressed the formation of new T cells. But both of these drugs tended to shut down the entire immune system. They left the patient as vulnerable to opportunistic infections and cancers* as someone with Aids would be. Cyclosporine, by contrast, seemed only to affect the signalling mechanisms connected to the T-cell receptor, the TCR. It stopped T-cell activation, but it didn't kill T cells, and it left other parts of the immune system – macrophages, monocytes, natural killer cells, antibody-spewing B cells – functioning. A patient taking only cyclosporine, say, for a liver transplant, actually had some ability to fight infection.

The ads Sandoz ran in the medical journals therefore proclaimed, above the image of the stick-figure skydivers falling through space: 'The most significant immunologic contribution to transplantation in the last 20 years.'

Sandoz was running a trial of cyclosporine as a preventative of GVHD, there at the Hutchinson Center, and wanted to compare a course of cyclosporine that started one day pre-transplant with one that started one day post-transplant. Carl June had put Maria

---

* Cancerous cells are thought to arise relatively often in the body, as a result of normal, random – or toxin or virus-caused – mutations in cellular DNA. A healthy immune system, it is believed, will generally wipe these cells out before they become tumours.

Morderas on cyclosporine one day pre-transplant, and she got a dose every day, the milky, castor-oil-based stuff coming down into her arm from a small clear plastic IV bag over her bed. Maria at least didn't have to take it orally. The oral solution tasted so foul that lab monkeys in animal trials fought their handlers tooth and claw, screeching and spitting and pissing, to avoid having so much as a teaspoonful of that milky, castor-oily poison scorch their gullets.

The days passed, and while the transplanted marrow cells established themselves amid the ruins of Maria's irradiated body, the delayed effects of the radiation became more pronounced. Her hair fell out completely. Her red blood cells, as they reached the limits of their useful lives, were not replaced by new blood cells – she didn't yet have blood-cells of her own – and so she received transfusions of red blood cells and platelets daily. Her gastrointestinal tract was still swollen and red, and the diarrhoea continued. And the pain, throbbing up now and then from beneath the morphine, was worse than ever.

Some time in the third week after the transplant, tests of Maria's blood showed that she now had some white blood cells. The donated marrow had established itself and had started to pump out life. She had reticulocytes now, and monocytes, and normal, non–cancerous granulocytes, and B cells that could make antibodies. And she had T cells.

A few days later a nurse noticed that the skin on Maria Morderas's hands and feet had begun to redden. As if she had had a bad sunburn. When Carl June saw this his heart sank. He knew this could be the beginning of graft versus host disease. T cells, for some reason, tended to make their first successful attacks in the skin, especially the skin of the hands and feet.

June and his colleagues ran some tests to rule out other causes – a reaction to one of the IV medicines, for example. Meanwhile the reddening of Maria's feet and hands worsened, and the skin there began to die and peel off. The results from skin biopsies came back, and it was clear that graft versus host disease had started. Cyclosporine, the miracle drug, had failed to prevent it.

June increased the dosage of cyclosporine, and now added prednisone in a further attempt to shut down Maria's new immune system, to curtail the marauding T cells her marrow was spawning. Time, he knew, was against him. Shutting down the T cells meant shutting off her immune system again. And she needed to have an immune system, even in the sterile environment of the isolation ward. Over time, over weeks and months in this situation, all the DNA viruses that lay dormant in a person's cells – herpes viruses, Epstein-Barr viruses, cytomegaloviruses; you might not know you have them, but you do – all these would stir and wake (hey, the coast is clear) and gradually shift from dormant mode into lethal, infect-everything mode.

June let up on the prednisone, and the marrow started up again, and the T cells came back, but they started attacking Maria's body again. The liver too was an early target of T cells in GVHD. And Maria's liver, under assault from her brother's donated T cells, began to fail. Her skin turned yellow with jaundice. June pumped her with prednisone again. And the T cells, snarling, fell away again. But now the viruses came out. An infection – cytomegalovirus – swelled her lungs with pneumonia. This was 1984; no drug effective against cytomegalorins had been invented yet.

Her liver almost dead, her lungs and other organs failing, her body now hooked to a respirator and draped with tubes and monitors inside the isolation ward, Maria Morderas slipped into a coma and died. She had lasted about three months after receiving her bone-marrow transplant. When it ended her family stood around her, husband and children, in gowns and masks and gloves. Only when she had died were they able to touch her.

Carl June wept with them. This was new for him. He felt that he was not yet a real oncologist, a hardened veteran of the cancer wars, with all the emotional barriers. He wept with Maria Morderas's family and then he wept alone and afterwards he went home to his own wife, and told her he had lost another one. Carl June did not know – he was not prone to premonitions – that in twelve years his wife would be diagnosed with metastatic ovarian cancer, and he would have to watch as she began much the same ordeal that Maria Morderas had had to endure, the ordeal of near-death.

10

The Secret Handshake

When the Sandoz Company advertised cyclosporine as 'the most significant immunologic advance in transplantation in the last twenty years', they were, in fact, not guilty of hyperbole. Most transplant surgeons would have agreed that cyclosporine was the best new drug in transplantation. Thanks largely to the Sandoz drug, many more transplants would be made possible, and the patients who received them would generally live longer. Cyclosporine, over the next decade, would bring transplant surgery almost to the point where one could call it routine medical practice.

But that didn't mean that cyclosporine made transplants easy, or free of complications. Cyclosporine was definitely not a miracle drug. Patients literally had a taste of that reality whenever they swallowed a teaspoonful or – later, when the pill version was available – popped a pinkish-brown capsule into their mouths. The awful skunk-spray taste warned, accurately, of vicious toxicity. Cyclosporine was particularly damaging to a patient's kidneys, but it was also toxic to the liver, and could cause an untreatable form of high blood pressure. And, like prednisone before it, cyclosporine had to be taken for a long time after a transplant, perhaps for ever, leaving the body highly vulnerable to infections, and cancers, especially B-cell lymphomas.

The drug also had problems with efficacy, which is to say, a patient often survived all those side-effects only to die when her immune system somehow overcame the drug and rejected her new organ. Or, in the case of bone-marrow transplant, when her new immune system overcame the drug and began rejecting the rest of her body.

For bone-marrow transplants cyclosporine would end up being

almost no advance at all over previous drugs. BMT patients were especially vulnerable to infections, and thus had to be given high doses of certain antibiotics which also were toxic to kidneys. The additional kidney toxicity from cyclosporine – a toxicity that was hard to judge in advance from the dose or even from bloodstream levels of the drug – could cause irreversible kidney failure. And even if it didn't, cyclosporine appeared not to have a great effect against graft versus host disease, the major complication of BMT surgery.

Carl June wondered why that was the case. Graft-versus-host-disease was a classic T-cell disease. A drug like cyclosporine, a drug whose claim to fame was that it stopped T-cell activation, should have been perfect against GVHD. But it wasn't. However effective cyclosporine had been against T-cell activation in the test tube, or in mice, it wasn't working nearly as well where it counted: in the bodies of humans.

And nobody knew why that should be. And nobody knew, really, why cyclosporine did succeed at stopping T-cell activation in the test tube. Even the biochemists at Sandoz, who had found cyclosporine by screening a massive collection of peptides found in funguses, didn't have much of a clue.

The truth was that immunology had long been a kind of *terra incognita* within medicine, a great black hole of confusion and ignorance. Even by the laggardly standards of medical science in general – compared to, say, rocket science, or theoretical physics – immunologists were forced with unusual frequency to admit that they didn't know what was really going on. Even today, at the turn of the millennium, one can go into three different immunologists' offices with the same medical history and come out with three different diagnoses and prescriptions, one doctor swearing by interferon gamma, another by Interleukin-2, the third by a mysterious blood-letting device known as a photopheresis machine – all of them swearing with the fervor of old time patent-medicine salesmen.

Twenty years ago immunologists at least were more humble. They knew that they knew next to nothing. They had not yet isolated and sequenced the TCR, the T-cell receptor, probably the most important protein in all of immune cell biology. They knew that it probably existed, but they had not found it. They did not even know for certain how the TCR bound to an antigen and caused a

T cell to become activated. Was it just as simple as that – stick an antigen in the TCR's paw, and watch the T cell explode into action? Or were other receptors involved? They didn't know!

Think how primitive that was. Pioneer 10 already had passed the planet Uranus, and soft grey moondust had softened the footprints of Neil Armstrong in the Sea of Tranquility, and the space shuttle had flown dozens of missions, and physicists were modelling the space-time warpage around black holes a million light years away – you could go on and on counting achievements in other areas – and meanwhile immunologists still knew hardly anything about the subject it was their job to understand.

This level of ignorance persisted until about the time Maria Morderas lay dying from her brother's 'well-matched' T cells.

The new tools of molecular biology, developed in the late seventies and early eighties, had given immunologists a better ability to isolate and sequence genes and their proteins. And with those tools the TCR was finally found in 1984; the TCR gene, immunologists noted, was always slightly different from one T-cell clone to another. They knew it had to be, because the TCR itself was always specific for a particular antigen. It also was discovered that a given T cell did not simply activate when its TCR locked on to its corresponding antigen. The antigen had to be cradled within a larger protein, an MHC protein (MHC stood for 'major histocompatibility complex') that stuck out from another cell, an 'antigen-presenting cell'. On the T cell side, the receptor situation was also complex – and as complex as I might make it seem here, I am still grossly simplifying the situation: a bundle of T-cell receptors including the TCR, a support receptor known as CD3, and another receptor dubbed CD4 (or CD8, for another class of T cells) fastened to the antigen-presenting cell's MHC, the TCR having a special little feeler that groped around, hoping to fasten to the antigen that the MHC bore in its grip. Imagine two portly, blind, but many-armed gentlemen bumping into each other on the street. 'Mr APC! Good day, sir!' 'Officer T cell! Very pleased to see you!' And exchanging handshakes – one with one arm, holding the little antigen in his palm ('I think you should feel this, Officer') the other simultaneously holding out three arms, three hands, the central hand feeling, with several agile and dozen-jointed fingers, for the antigen. Perhaps the antigen would fit snugly in this odd TCR grasp ('Yes, indeed, sir; you were right to bring this to my attention'), but perhaps the groping fingers would find nothing of interest ('Not my responsibility, sir, but thank you all the same').

MHC proteins appeared on virtually all cell types and they were always the same for a given person. The set of MHC proteins you possessed largely defined who you were, immunologically. And certainly the MHC situation was relevant to transplant rejections. One of the things that happened when a piece of foreign tissue was placed in a host's body – a kidney, for example, from a mismatched donor – was that T cells in the host body eventually encountered cells from this foreign tissue. A host T cell when it bumped into one of these cells would attempt the usual handshake, holding onto the other cell's MHC proteins and feeling around for an antigen.

Now, if this other cell was not 'foreign', if it was 'self', a part of the body's own tissue, and if it was not bearing any antigen to which the T-cell receptor was sensitive, then the T cell would go peacefully on its way ('Not my responsibility sir . . .'). But if this cell was foreign, the differentness of its MHC proteins would feel, to the properly equipped T cell, like a combination of self MHC and foreign antigen. And the T cell would go into battle mode ('Yes, indeed, sir, you were right to bring this to my attention – and now I shall have to kill you, sir'). It would treat the foreign cell more or less as it would treat a self cell infected and subverted by a foreign virus. ('I see that whatever your origins you are at present genetically unrelated to me, sir; I'm afraid that won't do, sir'.) The T cell would activate, spraying chemicals to work itself, and any T cells nearby, into a rage. And the T cell would make copies of itself, clones that is, and whenever a T cell in this clone grabbed and felt the oddly-shaped grip of such a foreign-MHC-bearing cell – 'I'm sorry to have to do this, sir!' – it would, chemically speaking, remove several sawed-off shotguns from within its capacious uniform and fire away.

That was the direct way T cells removed foreign tissue from the body. The indirect way – and the dominant way in transplant rejections – involved the usual presentation to T cells of antigen, in this case pieces of the transplanted foreign tissue, by self MHC on the surface of self cells. ('I thought you should feel this, Officer T cell . . .')

All that was for host versus graft disease. In graft versus host disease everything was the same except that the T cells were the real foreigners, and the tissue they were attacking, which to them was foreign, was not just some isolated organ but the entire body that surrounded them. ('Lovely country you have here, sir. Pity we shall have to destroy it'.)

Evolution, in other words, did not design T cells to mingle nicely with genetically different cells. It designed them to be genocidal monsters.

Cyclosporine, in the test tube, stopped the genocide. You could take T cells from one person, put them in a lab dish, and add T cells from a genetically mismatched person, and the mixed T cells would go into a frenzy of mutual attack. But if you added cyclosporine, all that would cease. Cyclosporine worked by interfering somehow with the way the three-armed TCR/CD3/CD4 complex coming from a T cell reacted to the MHC/antigen complex on an antigen presenting cell. It somehow blocked one of the chemical signals that ran from the TCR down into the deep bowels of the T cell, where battle-mode activation chemicals like Interleukin-2 were made. It blocked the sensation of that oddly-shaped foreign hand. It numbed the TCR's handshake.

Carl June and his colleagues wondered why this was not the case outside the test tube, in human bodies – in the doomed bodies of BMT patients like Maria Morderas. Cyclosporine numbed the TCR handshake, and that handshake was all that was needed for T-cell activation. Right? Or was some other, separate handshake involved in T-cell activation? A handshake that cyclosporine was not blocking?

When Carl June was not doing transplant operations, or attending patients on the oncology ward, he was working as a postdoctoral immunologist in a lab at Hutchinson. The lab was run by two of the world's leading transplant immunologists, John Hansen and E. Donnal 'Don' Thomas – who had worked on the world's first successful BMT, back in the early 1970s, and would later get a Nobel Prize for that.

At first June was placed on a small project with several other students, under the direction of Drs Paul Martin and Patrick Beatty. He found, soon enough, that it was a project that didn't particularly interest him – and in any case, he felt, there wasn't much he could do to help.

This is a dog project, he told himself.

Normally in such cases a postdoc had to grin and bear it, or just bear it. He had to do what the bosses told him to do, and go where they told him to go. But June's was a special case. His fellowship money was being paid not by the Fred Hutchinson Center, but by the US Navy, and that gave him some leverage. After three weeks he decided to quit. He told Hansen and Thomas he wanted to work on a new project. He wanted to investigate the reasons cyclosporine was so ineffective in preventing graft versus host disease. He wanted to find out if there was another receptor on T cells – another hand, another potential handshake – through which T cells involved in transplant rejection were being activated.

Hansen and Thomas were interested in the same question, and let Carl June go to work on this new project with Martin and Beatty. They also included a molecular biologist named Jeffrey Ledbetter, who worked across town, in Seattle, for a biotech company called Oncogen. Hansen had recently spent a year's sabbatical in the lab at Oncogen, and knew Ledbetter – and knew he too was intrigued by the cyclosporine conundrum.

So June and his colleagues began collaborating with Ledbetter. June did experiments at his own bench, in the lab at Hutchinson, and Ledbetter did his own experiments at Oncogen, and they talked about results, and suggested new experiments, and exchanged laboratory reagents, and so forth.

Both men, it turned out, were in the right place at the right time for this kind of investigation. A new tool for probing T-cell receptors had just been invented, and the Hansen/Thomas lab was one of the few labs in the world that possessed and knew how to use that tool.

The tool was the monoclonal antibody, whose invention was one of the cornerstones of biotechnology. Monoclonal antibodies were antibodies whose antigen-specific receptors (somewhat like antigen-specific TCRs on T cells) were all the same. The antibodies, in other words, were identical clones that had sprung from the same genes. Their receptors all bound to the same antigenic shape.

Monoclonal antibodies were produced by taking mice, injecting them with a group of foreign antigens (say, fragments of human T cells) and then removing their spleens a few weeks later when they had developed an immune reaction against these antigens. Immune cells known as B cells produced antibodies. Each B cell produced identical clones of a particular antibody specific for a certain antigen. When a mouse had been injected with an antigen, the B cells that produced antibodies specific for that antigen became activated and proliferated – much as T cells did when activated. In the weeks after a mouse had been injected with a foreign antigen, its B cell population – concentrated relatively heavily in its spleen – would become dominated by the B cell clones specific for the injected antigen.

Working at Cambridge University in the mid–1970s, Cesar Milstein and Georges Kohler discovered that they could harvest these B cells from mouse spleens and merge them, in laboratory dishes, with special cancerous, forever-dividing cells. In this way they could create hybrid cells ('hybridomas') each of which produced a single clone of antibodies indefinitely, like a little factory.

Because antibodies were so specific in what they bound to, they were invaluable as probes. They sought out and found a specific antigen in some laboratory dish, for example, sticking to it as tightly as anything could stick. You could biologically glue, to the tails of antibodies, radioactive molecules or molecules that would fluoresce under ultraviolet light, or some other little chemical signalling device that would tell you where the antibodies had bound. But before Milstein and Kohler's invention, a given test-tube full of antibodies could never be purified so that all the antibodies were identical clones that bound to the same thing. They were 'polyclonal' – they contained multiple clones that bound to multiple antigens. Therefore solutions of antibodies could never be made very specific as probes, at least not economically. But after Milstein and Kohler developed the idea of the hybridoma – for which they received the Nobel Prize and a big place in the history of science – it became possible to grow almost infinitely large numbers of a single, intensely specific clone of virtually any kind of antibody anybody might want.

A few years before Carl June had arrived at Hutchinson, John Hansen and Paul Martin had used the Kohler-Milstein technique to make a 'library' of monoclonal antibodies that bound to various human T-cell receptor proteins. Most of these T-cell receptor proteins were still part of the *terra incognita* of immunology. No one knew what they did, or what they looked like chemically. All anybody knew was what they weighed, because you could isolate them by weight on an electrophoresis gel.

One of the things that made an antibody especially useful for probing a T-cell receptor was this: Antibodies sometimes bound so tightly, so intimately, to receptors on cells that in the command post within the cell, the control panels lit up as if the receptor had just coupled with its natural 'ligand'. (The ligand for TCR/CD3/CD4, for example, was an MHC protein.) In other words the antibody successfully mimicked the special handshake the receptor normally got from another receptor on the surface of another cell. The antibody fooled the cell receptor into thinking that it, the antibody, was the ligand – and as a result the cell produced more chemicals, or began to make copies of itself, or whatever.

What June and Ledbetter intended to do was relatively straight-forward. They would take cultures of T cells, and add monoclonal antibodies from Hansen's anti-T-cell collection, each time checking to see how the T cell reacted to the new antibody. They wanted to find an antibody clone that would make T cells activate, inde-pendently of the TCR receptor channel. They wanted to find if there was a second channel, a second, secret handshake that T cells used to become activated – a handshake that wasn't blocked by cyclosporine.

Hansen and Martin, in developing their collection of monoclonals, had given each clone a simple numeric designation: 1.1, 1.2, 1.3, 2.1, 2.2, 2.3, and so on. June and Ledbetter decided to try almost all of them. They added monoclonals individually, and in combinations – 'mix 'n match', they called it – sometimes also adding cyclosporine or other drugs that blocked the TCR/CD3 channel.

June worked on this throughout the two years he spent at Hutchinson, dressed in his white lab coat, perched on his wooden stool, leaning over his 'bench' – his little space on the long hard shelf within the lab. Day after rainy Seattle day, when he could get away from patients and transplants and death, he pipetted solutions of monoclonal antibodies and other compounds into plastic dishes full of T cells. Then he ran tests on the T cells to see what their reactions would be.

And one day he found the thing he had been looking for.

It was a clone of T-cell-reactive antibodies that Hansen and Martin had given the stirring name of '9.3'. The third clone from the ninth hybridoma fusion dish.

The 9.3 clone bound to a T cell protein that had been dubbed Tp44 because its molecular weight was 44 kilodaltons.

Tp44 was almost a complete unknown in those days, but the 9.3 antibodies had begun to generate some interest. Around the time June and Ledbetter started their experiments, scientists in Germany reported that when the 9.3 antibodies were added to a T-cell activation culture they seemed to amplify the activation.

June and Ledbetter found that, plus something else: They found that 9.3 pushed T cells towards an activated state even when the TCR pathway was blocked with cyclosporine.

What that suggested was that the TCR pathway – the TCR handshake, which cyclosporine blocked – was not the only one that could activate a T cell. There was indeed another activation pathway involved. And that pathway involved a T-cell receptor called Tp44.

And nobody knew anything else about Tp44. But now Carl June, and soon everybody else in transplant immunology, understood that if you could block Tp44 on T cells, at the same time you blocked the TCR channel, you might be able to stop transplant rejection altogether. And if you could stop transplant rejection – as effectively, say, as you could stop a bacterial infection – then you would really have something. You would transform medicine, and how people lived. You would usher in a new age of spare parts.

11

The Ligand

Think about the concept of spare parts for a minute. Think about car parts. When the fuel pump in your Toyota goes bad, does your mechanic spend hours – assisted by coveralled, grease-spattered nurses – delicately cutting open the little fuel pump, painstakingly cleaning its innards with solvents, desperately trying to repair or shore up its blasted valves, its severed windings? Does he order up ten expensive tests of fuel pump function? Does he bring in some high-priced fuel pump specialist to lead the surgery?

No! He takes the whole damn thing out and sticks a new one in. All he has to know is where to cut and splice and bolt and unbolt. Cars don't swarm with little metal marauders that attack and destroy new spare parts. You can keep a car alive for ever, in principle, if you just keep replacing everything: fenders, hubcaps, engine, transmission, shocks, fuzzy dice. Replace every part in the entire car and it still retains its car-ness.

Of course I'm using the idea of car parts here just as an analogy with body parts. But when the problem of transplant rejection goes away, as it will some day – perhaps very soon, as you'll see – there may no longer be very much to separate the two.

The first thing to bear in mind is that when transplants become relatively easy, that is, uncomplicated by rejection and the need for immunosuppression, and uncomplicated by the shortage of spare organs, there won't just be more transplants. There will also be a qualitative change in medical thinking. Doctors who once would have repaired an organ will replace it instead. After all, who will care as much, in an age of spare parts, about all the things that can go wrong with, say, a human liver? Who will care about cirrhosis, and burrowing hepatitis viruses, and aflatoxin, and liver carcinomas?

Who will care about all the details of what can go wrong, when one can simply cut the old one out and put a new and healthy one in?

The same goes for parts of the body not usually thought of as transplantable. Suppose you discover that all the arteries around your heart and lungs are internally caked with atherosclerotic plaques. A heart attack, or a blood-spurting aneurysm, is just waiting for an excuse to happen. Do you throw away your Marlboros? Do you start popping aspirins and Mevacors? Do you cut your calories down to hallucination levels? Do you move to Hawaii and take up yoga and try to wash all the stress out of your life? No! You get your doctor-mechanic to cut out everything – arteries, heart, even both lungs if you want – and stick nice, pink, young ones in.

Or suppose you go to your doctor and he frowns and shows you the ominous shadows on the X-rays and says, well, sorry, but you have advanced metastatic cancer, and it's spread just about everywhere in your abdominal cavity.

No problem. Cut it all out. A radical evisceration – barely a day's work under the hood.

I may sound flippant here, continuing this car parts analogy when I talk about diseases that now cause so much misery and tragedy. But to me this is a good way to start imagining the gap, the huge gap, between (today) medicine as fixing-every-little-thing-until-it-fails-and-you-die and (tomorrow) medicine as a practice based mainly on large-scale replacement of damaged parts. That gap won't be crossed in a few months or years, but it will be made possible by only a few advances in technology, advances that are in the works now. I don't mean to sound flippant; I mean to sound optimistic.

Burn victims, now horribly disfigured, could get not just new and soft skin but whole new faces, bones and muscles and all. With advances in microsurgical techniques and nerve-regrowth drugs – and improvements in transplant technology will put pressure on scientists to make those advances – amputees could get new limbs, and not just decorative ones that have only a couple of nerves working and hang more or less limp, but completely functional ones.

With a better understanding of how neurons grow and connect, it will probably also become possible to inject new and young and healthy brain cells to replace older ones killed by Alzheimer's or Parkinson's or Lou Gehrig's disease or the ordinary decay of ageing. Who knows? – it may even become standard practice for people, for you, periodically to go to your neurotransplant mechanic for 'brain-matter replacement therapy', losing older and less desirable areas of memory (cut that dying grey stuff out) in exchange for infusions of virgin brain matter that can be more easily imprinted by new experience. You will retain a certain wisdom, from the old memories that remain, but your outlook will be fresher now, more youthful, no longer narrowed by the limits of your cranium, by the hardened neuronal networks of elderliness.

Wild daydreams like these had probably never afflicted the mind of Peter Linsley. His main concern, scientifically anyway, was cancer.

Linsley was employed at Oncogen, the biotech firm in Seattle where Jeff Ledbetter worked, and he ran a small project to study cell growth factors. The idea was to see whether these growth factors, chemicals with names like oncostatin, could be influenced to slow down or shut down the growth of tumour cells. It was important work. Cancer was an important disease.

But the truth was, Linsley didn't want to work on oncostatin any more. He was bored. He wanted to do something new.

Linsley walked into Jeffrey Ledbetter's office one day in 1989. The two men had sixth-floor offices next to one another, with windows looking soothingly out over the waterfront of central Seattle, right there off First Avenue. Linsley, then in his late thirties, was a dark-haired, somewhat serious-looking biochemist from Alabama, with large square-rimmed glasses and a soft Alabama accent. He had come out to Seattle a few years before from a postdoctoral slot in icy Toronto. Ledbetter was a bushy-haired fellow from Little Rock, Arkansas, but he'd been on the west coast a long time, loved Seattle. He was older than Linsley by a few years, but seemed always to have that bushy-haired youthful look about him.

Well, Jeff, said Linsley, I'm bored. I'm looking for something new. And Ledbetter thought about it and said, You might want to work on CD28.

What's CD28? wondered Linsley.

Ledbetter told him.

CD28 was the new term for Tp44. Four years had passed now since Ledbetter had done those cyclosporine experiments with Carl June. June, now a lieutenant commander, was back doing transplant operations at the Navy Medical Center in Maryland. The work that he and Ledbetter had done on Tp44 and cyclosporine had been published, after a long delay and many further experiments, in the journal *Molecular and Cellular Biology* in 1987. Papers were now pouring out on the subject.

A workshop that periodically convened to give some order to T-cell biology nomenclature had decided to give Tp44 a CD designation in 1986. CD was an old acronym that stood for 'cluster of differentiation', which just meant a cluster of cell stuff that separated out in similar groups when you fixed it with antibodies and flung it through a centrifuge and spread it out on a gel. Something that weighed 44 kilodaltons separated out together, and now it was being studied, so it needed a CD name. The CD28 slot had simply been available, like an unused phone number.

In the following decade dozens more CDs would be christened, as it became clear that the T cell was a bloated monster with more than a hundred kinds of arms, each with its own special handshake.

Virtually all of those handshakes, all of those multifarious Kamasutran methods of coupling, would be less interesting than the one in which CD28 took part. Yet the pace of work on that molecule, and its own special handshake, had been very slow for a while. CD28's molecular weight of about 44 kilodaltons was also the weight of certain MHC proteins found on virtually all cells in the body. That meant that the usual protein-isolation techniques – which depended on separating proteins by molecular weight – could not be used. CD28 could not practically be separated from ubiquitous MHC proteins.

These, however, were special days in immunology, as they were in all biology. The just-invented tools of biotechnology were spreading among the laboratories of the world, spawning new discoveries, new tools, new ways of thinking about and manipulating proteins and nucleic acids.

In 1987, at Massachusetts General Hospital, the molecular biologists Brian Seed and Alejandro Aruffo forged a handy protein-isolation tool that enabled scientists to get a better grip on CD28 and many other proteins.

Seed and Aruffo made history simply by combining the two fundamental tools of biotechnology. One of those tools was the monoclonal antibody. The other was the technique of recombinant

DNA expression, by which discrete genes could be inserted into cells and made to mass-produce their corresponding proteins.

CD28 was one of the first proteins the two scientists targeted with their new technique. I am going to simplify the complex reality of what Seed and Aruffo did, but not drastically: Seed and Aruffo started with a 'library' of separate DNA fragments that had been taken from the nuclei of T cells. These fragments, they knew, contained genes that coded for various T-cell proteins. No one had any idea what the proteins were, but Seed and Aruffo knew at least that CD28 would be one of these proteins.

Now, Seed and Aruffo used recombinant DNA technology to snap these T-cell DNA fragments, one by one, into groups of cells in laboratory culture dishes. In each dish, the culture of genetically implanted cells began to produce one particular type of T cell protein. Imagine a laboratory bench covered with hundreds of little plastic cell-culture dishes. Each expressed a different T-cell protein. Seed and Aruffo's job was to find the one that expressed CD28.

This was where the monoclonal antibodies came in. Seed and Aruffo took the anti-CD28 antibodies Carl June and Jeff Ledbetter had used in their experiments in Seattle – the antibody clone designated 9.3 – and chemically fastened little fluorescent tags to their tails. Then they sprinkled these fluorescent anti-CD28 antibodies on all the cultured cells, rinsed the cells to wash away antibodies that weren't specifically clinging to CD28, and lastly checked each group of cells for fluorescence, to find the one – the one expressing CD28 – to which the antibodies still clung.

Seed and Aruffo found such a dish (glowing bright with fluorescence under an ultraviolet blacklight) where the little anti-CD28 antibodies had stuck fast to cells. Now all they had to do was go back to their T-cell DNA library to look up the genetic fragment they had implanted in the cells in that glowing dish. They knew that that DNA fragment contained the CD28 gene. And knowing that, they could sequence the CD28 gene, working out the exact order of nucleic acids it contained. In turn they could use the CD28 gene – snapping it again into cells – to produce large quantities of purified CD28 protein in laboratory cell cultures.

With Seed and Aruffo's publication, later that year, of their 'expression cloning' of CD28, the field of CD28 studies began to get crowded. Now that CD28's sequence and structure were known, now that it could be produced easily in the lab, work could speed along towards the next big questions: how did CD28 – when something pressed its button – stimulate T-cell activation? And what was it out there in nature that pressed its button? What, in the vernacular of cell biology, was its ligand, the thing to which it tied itself? What chemical, or protein attached to another cell, touched it and made it shout down into the innards of the T cell: Battle stations! Activate!

No one knew. And everybody wanted to know. On the other hand, even if one didn't know the ligand, one might be able to block CD28 itself, and that would be something. If one could put a cork into CD28 – at the same time one stopped up the TCR pipe with cyclosporine – then perhaps the problem of organ transplant rejection would finally go away, or at least be greatly ameliorated. An effective CD28-corker might really deserve the label of 'wonder drug'.

But how to block CD28? The 9.3 antibodies certainly clung to CD28, but they did precisely the opposite of what a good CD28 blocker should do. Instead of blocking the signal, they transmitted an artificial one. They themselves pushed the T cell toward activation mode. To block the CD28 signal, it seemed, it might be better to block that ligand out there in the immune system that was sending the signal to CD28 in the first place. But again, no one knew what that ligand was.

And all this Jeff Ledbetter told Peter Linsley, as the two men sat in Ledbetter's office looking out over Elliot Bay.

Linsley thought about it, and decided it seemed like a good challenge. He knew almost nothing about immunology, of course. He knew, in fact, about as much as Ledbetter had just told him. But what the hell?

One of the nice things about working for a big company, contrary to the stereotypes, was that it allowed a scientist this kind of freedom. He could decide to do something, and then, more or less, could just start doing it. Oncogen and its parent company, Bristol Myers, were paying the bills. There were no grant proposals to write, no grant boards of curmudgeonly NIH-appointed professors to placate. And so Linsley, letting his technicians continue their work on oncostatin and other cancer growth factors, simply rolled up his sleeves and began to work, alone, on the mystery of CD28's ligand. The mystery whose solution might usher in the new medical age of spare parts.

Linsley had one clue that seemed to narrow his search for the ligand. As Seed and Aruffo had noted, the structure of CD28 suggested that it was not a receptor for some free-floating immune chemical – some cytokine – as, for example, the receptor CD25 was for interleukin-2. It was not the special button that a cytokine pressed to make a T cell do something. It looked instead like a receptor that had been designed to couple with a receptor sticking out from the surface of some other cell. CD28, in other words, was one part, one terminal, of some direct, cell-to-cell signalling pathway.

With this in mind Linsley began to work on CD28, and he worked long hours, and the months went by, through Seattle's wintry rains and summer droughts. He had a number of ideas about what the CD28 ligand might be – perhaps this or that molecule on other T cells, or on other cells in the body – but none of these ideas panned out.

One day Linsley decided to try his hand at cell-adhesion assays. In layman's terms: he would put genetically modified cells that expressed CD28 (sprouting CD28 from their surfaces, that is) in a series of dishes, and then would add another cell type to each dish to see which cell type stuck to the CD28-expressing cells. Once he had isolated the cell type that stuck best to the CD28-expressing cells, he would do further experiments to see which protein on those cells was actually binding to CD28.

This cell adhesion idea had logic to it. On the other hand, cell adhesion assays were generally very messy. Sometimes receptors on cells bound, weakly, to things they weren't supposed to bind to. Sometimes receptors in these artificial lab-dish systems took on the wrong shape, and didn't bind to other receptors as tightly as they should have. Linsley couldn't even be sure that the CD28 proteins his test cells expressed were functionally the same as natural CD28 proteins.

In any case, with the feeling that he might simply be flailing around in the dark, wasting his employer's money, Linsley did his cell adhesion assays.

He eventually found a cell type known as the T51 lymphoblastoid line that seemed to stick best to the CD28-expressing cells. T51 cells were a type of cancerous, immortal cell useful for laboratory work. They were related to B cells, the cells that produced antibodies. Linsley fooled around with other cell types, including inactive and activated B cells from mice. In the end he concluded that whatever it was that fastened tightly to CD28 in nature was probably found on activated battle-mode B cells. In other words, CD28's ligand was a protein expressed on the surface of activated B cells, and might be the signal by which activated B cells rallied T cells to become activated as well.

Linsley remained doubtful about all this, but he kept going. He took a collection of monoclonal antibodies that bound to various immune cell proteins, and started adding the monoclonals to his cell adhesion assays. The idea was to see which clone of antibodies would block the B cells' tight embrace of the CD28-expressing cells.

One monoclonal antibody worked well at this. It was a monoclonal that had been raised against a B-cell protein known as B7. Little was known about B7. It hadn't even received a CD designation yet.*

But Linsley now began to think that B7 might be what he'd been looking for: the ligand, on B cells as it happened, that bound to CD28 on T cells.

Linsley still was sceptical. This B-cell/T-cell interaction seemed too weird to be true. But that was where the trail led, and he followed. A year and a half had passed since he had started work on this area, and it was now 1990. A recent development meant that he could take a definitive last step. Another group of researchers, using the Seed/Aruffo technique, had just cloned the B7 gene. So Linsley borrowed the B7 gene from them, snapped it into a cell line, and now had cells that expressed only B7. He took these B7-expressing cells, tagged them with radioactive molecules, and added them to a dish of the special cells expressing CD28. If these two groups of cells bound tightly to each other, resisting the pressures of rinsing, then he could be fairly certain that B7 was the long-sought ligand for CD28.

In this particular cell adhesion assay the bottom of the plastic lab dish was covered with a layer of the CD28-expressing cells. The B7 cells were added to the top of this layer, and then rinsing was done to see if they would slide away or stick around. After the rinsing, and before he placed a gamma-ray counter atop the dish to record the energetic photons from the little radioactive tags on the B7 cells,

---

* B7 was so-called because it was the seventh B-cell structure identified by a lab at the Dana Farber Cancer Research Institute in Boston.

Linsley simply peered at the dish of double-layered cells through a stereo microscope.

What he saw reminded him of a tick he had once seen in his childhood, one day as he wandered in the swampy Alabama woods. The tick was big and round and pale, engorged with the blood of some punctured mammal. The cells in the dish looked like that, so passionately had they fastened to one another.

Linsley leaned back and let out a rebel yell. The others in the lab and in the nearby hallway came running.

12

The Blocker

In time Linsley and others would discover that B7 was expressed on a variety of activated cells, not just B cells. It was also expressed on bacteria- and virus-gobbling macrophages, and epithelial cells. These kinds of cells, these antigen-presenting cells, presented MHC-plus-antigen to T cells, at the same time they presented B7. B7 was a big red hand that had been reaching around to shake that secret handshake with CD28 while immunologists, peering down through their microscopes, had been busy watching the TCR/MHC interaction. They should have been looking at CD28 too, and now they were. CD28 was the portal for a major activation channel, and blocking it, jamming it, by tinkering with it or with B7, could be the key to making tissue transplants easy.

But – how to block the CD28-B7 channel? What kind of drug would do it?

For a few years Jeff Ledbetter had been hearing about work at Genentech Co., the big biotech house down in South San Francisco. Scientists at Genentech had reported initial success with so-called 'fusion proteins': proteins tagged with the tails of antibodies.* Those tails were easy to grab and manipulate in the test-tube. They made proteins connected to them easier to study. They also made such proteins more stable in the body. The existence of the antibody tail somehow kept a protein to which it was attached from being digested or metabolized away too quickly.

---

* Antibodies, generally speaking, are Y-shaped proteins. The arms at the top of the Y (the Fab fragment) form the antigen-specific binding region. The stem of the Y (the Fc fragment) serves as both a stabilizer and a signalling region to other elements of the immune system, such as complement proteins.

Genentech was already developing a drug based on a fusion protein. It was called CD4Ig. CD4 was that receptor molecule found on certain T cells. The '-Ig' part was the anitbody tail, 'Ig' being an abbreviation of 'immunoglobulin', a general term for antibody-like proteins.

Knowing that the Aids-causing virus, HIV, infiltrated cells primarily through the T-cell CD4 receptor, to which it bound tightly, Genentech researchers had developed the free-floating CD4Ig molecule as a blocker of HIV infection. CD4Ig smothered, like millions of barnacles, all the parts of HIV virions that could bind to CD4 on T cells. It worked wonderfully in the test tube.

Ledbetter, talking it over with Linsley, decided that the same logic could be applied to B7 and CD28. They could flood the body with little copies of CD28 – as CD28Ig – which would coat B7 proteins on antigen-presenting cells, thus preventing the B7 proteins from coupling with the real CD28 receptors on T cells . . . thus preventing the activation of T cells. Thus preventing transplant rejection, among other things.

Linsley, working now with a lab technician named Bill Brady, made Ig fusion proteins based on CD28, and began to study their interactions with B7-expressing cells in the test tube. How tightly would they bind together? How good would they be as a blocker of T-cell activation?

The surprising answer, which Linsley and Brady learned after several months of painstaking, stop-start work, was this: CD28Ig worked not very well at all.

It bound to B7 only weakly. Whereas to block B7 in the body effectively, Linsley knew, CD28Ig proteins would have to cover a large fraction, probably a majority, of the B7 receptors on antigen-presenting cells in the body. Doing that with a reasonable dose of CD28Ig meant that the CD28Ig would have to bind very tightly, very specifically, to those B7 receptors. But it just didn't. With such a weak binding ability for his imagined wonder drug, Linsley knew he would have to virtually saturate a transplant patient's bloodstream with it – something that would be impossibly expensive, to say nothing of the probable toxicity.

Linsley and Ledbetter soon saw that Genentech scientists were beginning to confront the same problem. Though their CD4Ig product worked like a charm in the test tube, it worked poorly in clinical trials. The doses that might have been effective were impractically high.*

Linsley's research might have reached a dead end, right there with CD28Ig, but one day he received a fateful phone call from Craig Thompson, an immunologist then at the Howard Hughes Institute at the Unwersity of Michigan.

Thompson recently had quit the Navy, where for a time he had done postdoctoral work alongside Carl June at the Hutchinson Center in Seattle. He had been involved in the CD28 work a long time; he and his wife Tullia Lindsten had even been co-authors, with Jeff Ledbetter, on Carl June's original paper about the 9.3 antibodies and cyclosporine. So he knew the CD28 story. And he knew Linsley wasn't having much success getting CD28Ig to bind to B7.

As Thompson explained to Linsley, his wife Tullia had just come back from a conference in Israel. At the conference she has spoken about the CD28 work, noting among other things that the DNA sequence data on the mysterious T-cell molecule suggested that it was, evolutionarily, from the same family as immunoglobulin molecules. A French researcher, Pierre Golstein, had come forward with an interesting observation: years before, Golstein and his team had sequenced some genes from killer T cells – cells known more formally as cytotoxic T lymphocytes, or CTLs – and one of those genes, coding for a CTL surface protein Golstein dubbed CTLA4, also looked like it belonged to the immunoglobulin family.

Lindsten mentioned this to her husband when she got back to the States, and together they put the sequences for CD28 and CTLA4 through the computer. They found that the sequence for CTLA4's gene was indeed remarkably similar to the sequence for the CD28 gene. That was very odd. But whatever the reason for it, it suggested that CTLA4 might also bind to B7.

Thompson told Linsley all this over the phone. Why not try a

---

* Genentech and its competitors eventually abandoned work on CD4Ig. In addition to the problem of getting enough CD4Ig into a patient's blood economically, scientists also confronted the fact that HIV could infect cells through receptors other than CD4.

fusion protein based on CTLA4? he suggested. See how well it binds to B7.

Later, when there was a lawsuit over all this, Linsley and Ledbetter would say they saw little reason why CTLA4 should work. CD28 was the evolved ligand for B7. The idea that there would be another T-cell molecule that bound even better to B7 was just bizarre. Why should B7 be bound more tightly by some other protein than by the ligand evolution had apparently designed for it?

Nevertheless, Linsley followed Thompson's suggestion. He had nothing better to do. He fused the tails of antibodies to recombinant CTLA4 proteins, forming a fusion protein he called CTLA4Ig. Then he began to run experiments to see how well CTLA4Ig bound to B7.

The key instrument Linsley used in this series of experiments was known as a flow cytometer. About two feet wide, a foot deep, and eighteen inches high, it squatted on a benchtop at one end of the lab. Within the machine, cells flowed through a narrow channel, one by one, bathed in blue-green light from an argon laser. An optical detector registered the intensity of fluorescence emitted by the laser-illuminated cells. The idea of this machine was to take antibodies or other proteins, tag them with fluorescent molecules, and add them to a dish of cells. The dish of cells would then be rinsed to remove the proteins that had not bound anywhere. Then the cells would be put through the fluorescence-measuring channel. The higher the fluorescence of the cells moving through the channel, the higher the avidity with which the fluorescence-tagged proteins had stuck to the cells.

Linsley took cells that had been transfected with the B7 gene, and were therefore expressing the B7 protein. He put them in a laboratory dish. Then he added CD28Ig molecules that had been tagged with tiny fluorescent molecules. Then he rinsed everything, to wash away CD28Ig molecules that hadn't bound to the B7-expressing cells. Then he put the rinsed cells through the flow cytometer. The more the cells glowed as they passed through the detection channel, the higher the signal on the oscilloscope.

Linsley watched as this first batch of cells passed through the cytometer. The signal was high, but not as high as it could be, signi-fying that the fluorescence-tagged CD28 molecules had bound to the

B7 cells with only moderate intensity. That he knew already. What he wanted to do now was compare this result with CTLA4Ig.

Linsley added the next batch of cells. These were B7 cells that had been soaked with fluorescent CTLA4Ig, then rinsed as before. If the signal was lower this time, as Linsley expected, it would mean that CTLA4 bound even less tightly to B7 than CD28 did.

But as the first cells began to pass through the cytometer, the oscilloscope trace jumped to the top of the screen. The CTLA4Ig molecules had bound to B7 more tightly than CD28 had. Many times more tightly.

It was around 6 p.m., and most of the others in the lab, including Jeff Ledbetter, had left for the day. Linsley had never bothered Ledbetter at home before. This time, picking up the phone, he did.

The full significance of CTLA4Ig was still far from being understood, but already one thing was clear. The molecule CTLA4, which occurred naturally – for some reason – on the surfaces of T cells (not just killer T cells, it turned out) was a *second* evolved ligand for B7. It seemed actually to have been designed by nature as a blocker of the B7/CD28 T-cell activation channel.

When Linsley added CTLA4Ig to assays in which B7 would normally activate T cells (via CD28) T-cell activation was prevented – because B7 had been smothered by the little CTLA4Ig proteins. CTLA4Ig performed far better, in this role, than CD28Ig. CTLA4Ig was, in short, a surprise candidate and by far the best candidate for a drug that could block B7 and thus prevent transplant rejections.

Linsley's first paper on CTLA4 announced that it, like CD28, was a natural receptor for B7. The paper came out in the *Journal of Experimental Medicine* in late 1991. By then Linsley, heading a growing cadre of workers, had begun to do *in vivo* experiments with CTLA4Ig.

Along the way Linsley also loaned samples of the fusion protein to a group at the University of Chicago led by immunologist Jeffrey Bluestone. Bluestone, hearing about Linsley's initial results with CTLA4Ig, had written Linsley a long letter setting forth his ideas about experiments that could be done.

Bluestone did these experiments, and Linsley's group did their own experiments. These experiments were ambitious, and involved tests of CTLA4Ig in animals.

When the papers from the two labs were published, one after the other, in an issue of *Science* in May 1992, they sent a shock wave of excitement through the international network of immunologists. There was a full-page Research News story in *Science*, and there was plenty of secondary coverage in the popular press – including a prominent piece in the *Wall Street Journal*. Later Linsley would also be profiled in *Forbes*. It was no coincidence that these money-minded journals were interested. CTLA4Ig, it now appeared, was going to be one of the most important biotech drugs ever created.

In their experiments, Linsley's team had injected mice with two foreign antigens normally used to stimulate vigorous immune responses. These antigens were, first, sheep red blood cells, and second, haemocyanin proteins from a mollusc known as the keyhole limpet. Something about the antigenic shape of those proteins drove mouse immune systems into a rage of activity.

As expected, when the mice were injected with these antigens alone they developed frenzied immune reactions. But when CTLA4Ig was also given to the mice there was little or no immune reaction. CTLA4Ig had suppressed both T cell and antibody responses. Even when immunological storms were raging in mice injected with the antigens, CTLA4Ig, added later, substantially calmed the storm. Other data showed that CTLA4Ig had been both stable and non-toxic in the mice, suggesting that it would make an excellent drug in humans.

Impressive as they were, Linsley's results were outshone by Bluestone's. Led by postdoctoral student Debbie Lenschow, the Bluestone group had actually performed a transplant experiment, using CTLA4Ig to block rejection.

Lenschow and her colleagues had started by inducing a form of diabetes in mice – chemically destroying their pancreatic 'islet' cells, the ones that produce insulin. Then they had transplanted human islet cells into the mice. To a mouse's immune system, of course, human cells would normally be seen as foreign. The human cells would be attacked by the mouse's T cells in short order, and wiped out. And the mice untreated with CTLA4Ig quickly did lose their new islet cells to rejection, and died from lack of insulin. But all the mice treated with a high dose of CTLA4Ig kept their islet cells. CTLA4Ig had blocked the activation of the T cells that ordinarily would have killed the donated, foreign islet cells.

The strangest thing that Lenschow and her colleagues found was this: mice that had been successfully treated with CTLA4Ig at the time of transplant could later receive a second transplant from the same human donor, without the need for additional treatment with CTLA4Ig.

It was as if the first treatment with CTLA4Ig had somehow fooled the mouse's immune system into thinking, permanently, that the incoming islet cells – and all other cells from that same donor – were not 'foreign', but were instead 'self', a part of the host mouse. A single course of treatment with CTLA4Ig, in other words, apparently had induced permanent immunological 'tolerance' specifically to tissue from a given donor. No other drug had been given – no prednisone, no cyclosporine. The mouse immune system was intact; it could fight off infections; it could reject tissue from other donors. The only thing it couldn't do was attack tissue from the specific human donor who had provided the islet cells.

It all happened so quickly, so suddenly. Nevertheless there it was. Immunologists who had been toiling on the problem for years now looked blearily up from their lab benches. The dream – the old dream of trouble-free transplantation – was here.

In mice, at least.

13

The Grail

The induction of specific tolerance – tolerance to tissue from a specific donor, while the rest of the immune system stayed intact – had long been known as the 'Holy Grail' of transplant immunology. The reason was obvious: if you could induce specific tolerance to a desired antigen, you could not only transplant all kinds of tissue and organs relatively easily, without fear of rejection – you also could treat autoimmune disorders such as multiple sclerosis, which are caused when the immune system mistakenly attacks 'self' antigens, perceiving them as foreign.

The concept of specific tolerance – the idea that it was biologically possible – had started, more or less, with the British zoologist Peter Medawar in 1953.

Medawar had noticed around then, from the literature and from some preliminary experiments, that foetal and newborn animals seem much more tolerant of grafted foreign tissue than adults. Their immune systems, in other words, are much less likely to raise a fuss about an incoming transplant. To nail all this down Medawar and two of his lab scientists, Rupert Billingham and Leslie Brent, did a formal experiment.

They injected six foetal mice, still in their mother's womb, with cells from an adult mouse of an unrelated strain they termed the 'A-line'. Four days later, five of the injected mice were born healthy (the sixth had died in the womb). When the five mice had reached the age of eight weeks Brent and Billingham grafted skin from an A-line donor – the A-line skin was albino–pink, the hair very white – on to the backs of the five mice. Then the two men put the mice back in their cages.

Had the experiment been done in, say, adolescent mice instead of foetal/newborn mice, the grafts would have died and flaked off from rejection within about eleven days. That was what always happened; you could almost set your watch by it. But in these young mice, three of the five grafts had clearly 'taken' after eleven days. They had engrafted as if they had always belonged to their new mouse owner, even though they were noticeably pinker, their hair whiter.

Two and a half months later one of these three grafts slowly failed. But the other two kept on. Medawar, in his three-and-a-half page paper that appeared in *Nature* later that year, argued that the recipient mice had become specifically tolerant to the foreign antigens because they had been exposed to them before birth. Something about the foetal stage of development allowed this to happen.

Something . . . But what?

Immunologists struggled with this question for years, but got nowhere. The tools they had for investigating the immune system were just inadequate. The Grail constantly eluded their grasp.

There were theories about tolerance. The most compelling was developed decades later, when the origins and functions of T cells became clearer. This theory took note of the fact that T cells, after they emerged in prototype form (all immune cells emerged and differentiated from special marrow-based cells called stem cells), found their way to the thymus, a nut-sized organ below the neck. The thymus was a school where T cells were taught the difference between right and wrong. Or as one might say in America today, they were taught 'values'.

T-cell values were straightforward. First commandment: antigens normally found on cells in this body are OK. Second commandment: antigens not normally found on cells in this body are to be destroyed.

T cells that didn't obey this value system were not spanked or scolded. They underwent a process that came to be called 'clonal deletion'. That is to say, the clones that locked into self antigens were killed, or were switched into a special 'suicide mode' so that they soon dropped dead, or were somehow or other deactivated. All young T cells went into the thymus, but only the ones whose TCRs did not react to self-antigens came out.* In the thymus, you might say, the T-cell army removed

---

* Remember that TCRs occurred in great variety, to cope with the billions of potential foreign antigens that nature might throw at the body. The genes that coded for the TCR were different for every T-cell clone, thus every clone had its own unique TCR, its own special recognition device that locked on to a particular antigenic shape out there in nature. When a group of antigens, say, from a flu virus, entered the body in substantial numbers, the T-cell clones whose TCRs could fasten to those flu antigens became activated and multiplied. When the foe had been conquered, this bulging population of warriors went into a resting mode for months or years – able during this time to go immediately to battle mode – and only gradually died out.

from its ranks all the sociopaths and traitors, leaving only sane warriors programmed to kill foes.

Precisely how did the body determine which T cells floating through the thymus were sociopaths and traitors? Well, no one knew, but it was supposed that immature T cells in the thymus were simply exposed to an array of the more prominent antigens found in the self's body. Those T cells whose TCRs recognized those antigens (and thereby, perhaps, became activated and went into battle mode) were killed or switched off.

If you wanted to test this theory about thymic teaching you could do an experiment. You could take a young animal, animal one we'll call it, and inject cells from a genetically mismatched animal, animal two, into animal one's thymus. You could do that while animal one was a foetus, and its immune system was still forming. So T cells going through school in animal one's thymus would be exposed to the antigens from animal two, and those T cells that reacted against those foreign antigens would be removed from the ranks. The resulting immune system of animal one would therefore lack T cells that could react against animal two's antigens.

Some immunologists guessed that that was what had happened in Medawar's experiment: enough of the cells injected into the foetal mice had migrated to their thymuses and there had induced tolerance to the foreign antigens on the injected cells. And – perhaps – the cells had got into the thymuses of only three out of the five mice, which explained why the other two mice had rejected their subsequent grafts. And – again perhaps – the reason this didn't work in older mice was that they already had populations of mature T cells that had gone through thymus school and were circulating in their blood and hanging around in their lymph nodes. They already had T cells that could react against any foreign antigen. You would have to get rid of those mature T cells first, if you wanted to see any tolerance effect from injecting foreign antigens into the thymus.

Almost forty years after Medawar's experiment, in 1990, a transplant immunologist put this more advanced idea to the test. The immunologist, Ali Naji, was actually a full-time transplant surgeon at the University of Pennsylvania's Medical Center. He and his lab workers did a transplant experiment in mice, as Medawar had done, but this time they used mature mice.

First they effectively destroyed the T-cell population in one group of mice, the recipient group, using a monoclonal antibody that bound to the CD3 receptor on T cells. After that Naji's group injected the thymuses of the recipient mice with islet cells from a genetically mismatched donor group of mice. Then they waited for new T cells to filter through the thymuses of the recipient mice, this new population of T cells now – hopefully – lacking any clones that would attack the cells of donor mice.

After a few weeks, Naji and his colleagues tried the transplant. Using a chemical called streptozotocin, they killed the insulin-producing islet cells beneath the pancreases of the recipient mice. Now these mice had diabetes and would die without insulin-producing cells. So Naji and his group transplanted new islet cells from the donor group into the recipient group, the group that had just lost theirs. If the transplants 'took', the mice would live. If they were rejected, as they normally would be, the mice would quickly die from lack of insulin.

The mice lived. Their new islet cells were not rejected. Naji's paper on all this was published with fanfare in *Science*, and Naji, who already worked about sixteen hours a day doing pancreas and kidney transplant operations for desperate patients, was suddenly swamped with reporters' phone calls. Was this the end? reporters asked. Had Doctor Naji at last found the Grail of transplant immunology? Had he found the subtle switch that induced tolerance to tissue from a specific donor while leaving the rest of the immune system untouched?

Well, no. As other immunologists pointed out, the thymus played a greater role in the mouse immune system than it did in the more complex and advanced human immune system. In fact, as humans matured to adulthood, their thymuses wilted and wrinkled and shrank, like grapes turning into raisins. The thymus of an adult human was almost a vestigial organ, left behind by evolution but still hanging around, barely. Experiments with Naji's thymic-teaching method were never done in humans, because even rabbits and dogs, subjected to the Naji method in the years after the mouse experiment, failed to become tolerant to injected donor antigens.

Immunologists concluded that donor-specific tolerance in higher mammals, if it could be induced at all, would probably have to be induced somewhere other than the thymus. It would probably have to be induced by sending specific 'off' signals to mature T cells, not centrally in some organ such as the thymus but peripherally, out there on the arterial highways and lymphatic byways of the body. Until immunologists figured out how such peripheral tolerance worked, that part of the dark continent of immunology would remain dark.

Simplistically, the idea of peripheral tolerance was this: a T cell fresh from the thymus and circulating in the body, waiting for orders, could be put into one of two states depending on the signals it received from antigens and other cells.

One state, of course, was activation – battle mode. The other state was 'anergy' – inactivation. An anergic T cell, in effect, was one that had been handcuffed and muzzled. The key to transplant tolerance would be the signal that switched T cells into this anergic mode.*

Early in 1987, almost a year before Carl June's and Jeff Ledbeffer's paper on cyclosporine-resistant T-cell activation appeared, two NIH immunologists published the results of an anergy experiment in the *Journal of Experimental Medicine*. The immunologists, Marc Jenkins and Ron Schwartz, had used mouse spleen cells to present a powerful T-cell stimulating antigen (pigeon cytochrome c) to mouse T cells in a culture dish.

Normally the spleen cells worked well as antigen-presenting cells. They sucked up foreign antigens, presented them to T cells, and – boom – the T cells activated.

The catch here, in the Jenkins–Schwartz experiment, was that the antigen-carrying spleen cells were treated with a chemical called ECDI. Precisely what that chemical did to the spleen cells wasn't clear. But it did something. It modified spleen cell receptors, or tore them off. It did something that changed the signals coming from the spleen cells to the T cells. Because now the T cells, instead of becoming activated, or doing nothing, became specifically inactivated.

Those ECDI-modified cytochrome-carrying spleen cells could even be injected into mice, to prevent a big reaction when the mice were later inoculated with the cytochrome antigens. The modified

---

* Immunologists had been theorizing about a 'two-signal model' for T-cell activation since 1970, when the idea was proposed by Peter Bretscher and Mel Cohn in an essay in *Science*.

spleen cells specifically *switched off* the T-cell clones that normally would have been running around attacking cytochrome antigens.

What had ECDI done to those antigen-presenting cells to change, so drastically, the signals they sent to T cells?

That remained a puzzle for a while. But Jenkins and Schwartz and others had concluded by 1991 that there were probably two activation signals involved here. The antigen-presenting cell transmitted one activation signal through the antigen/MHC complex (which coupled with the TCR/CD3/CD4 complex on the T cell). That was known; it was an old idea. The newer idea was that the antigen presenting cell transmitted a *second* activation signal through some other receptor which bound to a corresponding receptor on the surface of a T cell. If the two signals were firing at the same time, the T cell would become activated. But, if the first, TCR-based signal was there but the second signal was missing – if the receptor that transmitted it had been suppressed or destroyed by ECDI or some other agent – then the T cell would switch to inactive, anergic mode.

Of course, while all this theorizing was going on, research on the T-cell receptor CD28 was proceeding at full speed. Scientists like Carl June and Peter Linsley and Jeff Ledbetter were finding that CD28 was a portal for a second, previously undiscovered T-cell activation signal. They were finding out about B7, too, the ligand on antigen-presenting cells that coupled with CD28 to transmit the activation signal.

Eventually the theorists, such as Jenkins and Schwartz, looked over and noticed what was happening and – Eureka! – realized that the B7/CD28 signal was the second signal they all had been theorizing about. The chemical ECDI, they understood now, had prevented the expression of B7 on the spleen cells in those experiments, thus preventing the second signal from being transmitted – which explained why the T cells had gone into anergic mode instead of battle mode.

With this sudden marriage of high theory and laboratory curiosity, other things became clear. Peter Linsley's CTLA4Ig hadn't just blocked a T-cell activation signal by blocking B7. It hadn't just put itself in the way of the normal T-cell activation channel. No, the absence of the B7 signal, in the presence of an antigen coupling with the T cell's TCR, actually constituted a separate powerful signal, which said to the T cell: Stop! Shut down! Go into anergic mode!

*   *   *

One question remained in all this, and that was the question of CTLA4. Remember, it was not some obscure peptide found in some exotic fungus, as cyclosporine was. It was not some complicated compound synthesized by a chemist in some smoke-spouting factory. It was a natural protein found in humans and other mammals. It was a receptor molecule that sprouted from the membranes of activated T cells.

What did it do? What was its function? Why had it evolved?

In the two or three years following Peter Linsley's paper describing the first mouse experiments with CTLA4Ig, the answers to these questions started to glimmer into awareness. One thing immunologists noticed was that there was hardly any CTLA4Ig on resting T cells, that is, pre-activated T cells. But when a T cell activated, something went on in the genes down below and, after about forty-eight hours, CTLA4 started to boil up from down there and pop out through the T-cell membrane. Suddenly the T cell was, relatively speaking bristling with CTLA4. And because CTLA4 bound so much better to B7 than CD28 did, it effectively blocked the B7 receptors on antigen-presenting cells from their attempts to couple with CD28. That, of course, pushed the T cell towards anergic mode.

CTLA4's function therefore seemed to be to rein in a T cell after it had been let loose for a couple of days of frenzied killing. Too much killing, after all, could result in too many unhelpful side-effects.* The gene for CTLA4 had probably started its life as a loose copy of the CD28 gene, plopping into a new position somewhere down the genome, and had then gradually evolved its braking, T-cell damping function. Scientists would soon find that people who lacked the proper form of CTLA4 on their T cells, for genetic reasons, seemed highly susceptible to autoimmune diseases. Their T cells, apparently, had a lot of 'on' switches, but the 'off' switches were broken.

The Grail glowed brightly, so low in the sky it seemed easily within reach.

---

* The chemicals produced by activated immune cells can cause widespread cellular damage as well as unpleasant symptoms of headache, muscle-ache, fever and nausea.

Immunologists recognized now that if a T cell encountered a foreign antigen, but failed to be stimulated simultaneously by its second activation signal, by B7 that is, it would switch off, perhaps for ever. If this occurred across the body, among T cells specific for a given antigen, the immune system would effectively become tolerant specifically to that antigen, but would otherwise be healthy and intact. And now, with CTLA4Ig, scientists had the power to block that second signal, to induce that tolerance to specific antigens.

Theoretical immunologists, ordinary immunologists, transplant immunologists, experimental transplant surgeons – all now exulted. They gathered at workshops and conferences to rejoice. Tolerance! The mechanism illuminated at last!

Already, by the time the Linsley and Lenschow papers were published, others had heard the news and were racing to expand the frontiers of knowledge about CTLA4Ig. Up in Michigan at the Howard Hughes Institute, Craig Thompson – who had first suggested to Peter Linsley that he make the CTLA4Ig fusion protein – had used the magic biotech drug in transplanting hearts between one rat species and another. In the year following those first CTLA4Ig papers in *Science*, Thompson and Linsley and Lenschow and others used the drug, in animals, to prevent transplant rejection, to stop graft versus host disease, and even to prevent autoimmune diseases.

It was clear to everyone that if such results could be repeated in humans, CTLA4Ig could be an enormous success commercially, transforming medicine in a way that few drugs had. Provided that the shortage of donor organs could somehow be overcome, whole areas of medical science would become de-emphasized in favour of transplant science. How much money CTLA4Ig would make its owners, no one knew – CTLA4Ig would create its own market as it made transplants routine throughout the world – but it would not have been at all wild to suggest eventual sales in the range of 10 billion dollars per year.

With this kind of wealth in prospect, it was not too surprising that a schism split CTLA4Ig researchers, a schism from either side of which was waged an intense, acrimonious competition.

It all stemmed, some said, from the corporate fate of Oncogen, the employer of Peter Linsley and Jeff Ledbetter. Oncogen had been bought by drug giant Bristol Myers in 1986, but for a few years had been left largely alone.

Then in 1989 Bristol Myers had merged with fellow colossus Squibb, forming the behemoth known as Bristol Myers Squibb (BMS). As part of the long restructuring that followed, the new conglomerate had swallowed Oncogen, firing many of its employees and turning its laboratory in downtown Seattle into the Bristol Myers Squibb Research Institute. The BMS culture was imposed on the Oncogen staff, and to those outside scientists who had been collaborating with Linsley and Ledbetter, it was as if an iron curtain had fallen – especially after it became clear that CTLA4Ig was a potential blockbuster drug.

At the University of Chicago, Debbie Lenschow and Jeff Bluestone were denied further access to CTLA4Ig. At the Naval Medical Research Institute in Maryland, Carl June was denied access to CTLA4Ig. At the Howard Hughes Institute in Michigan Craig Thompson – without whom Peter Linsley probably would not have invented CTLA4Ig – was also denied access to the fusion protein.

No one blamed Linsley or Ledbetter. The two scientists, it seemed, had been all in favour of collaboration and cooperation, having benefited greatly from it themselves. But the suits at BMS headquarters in New York apparently had ordered a cordon to be placed around the CTLA4Ig work, and that was that.

In response, Lenschow and Bluestone and June and Thompson and others began to rally around a rival to BMS: Repligen, a young Boston biotech house that had licensed the patent for an anti-B7 antibody and had also begun to make its own version of CTLA4Ig, a version with enough biological differences from the BMS version that it could at least force BMS to a patent court showdown – or possibly a large payoff. Craig Thompson, backed by Repligen, even filed a lawsuit against BMS, contesting that its CTLA4Ig patent was invalid because it did not include Thompson on the list of patentors.

The fight was not quite even. BMS was a Goliath, with assets to match those of a small country. Repligen was an unworthy David. Even before it reached a showdown with BMS it ran into the usual biotech house financial crisis – too many debts, too little cash from its flagship products – and in the mid 1990s it began to sell off assets. Its CTLA4Ig programme was picked up by one of its Boston neighbours, a biotech company called Genetics Institute.

But the fight went on, as scientific papers continued to be published about CTLA4Ig, and the drug neared its first trials in humans. And through all the acrimony and pulling of hair and lawsuits, through all the excitement about CTLA4Ig as the Holy Grail, the magical key to controlling immune reactions, an embarrassing fact began to emerge:

CTLA4Ig was not working.

Peter Linsley had glimpsed this from the beginning. In his first CTLA4Ig experiments, when he had injected mice with the drug to suppress reactions against two potent immunogens, he had noticed that suppression of the reaction did occur. But subsequent injections of these immunogens, in the absence of CTLA4Ig treatment, still brought about major immune reactions. In other words, tolerance had not been induced. It was there in his first paper in *Science*, in plain black and white: 'we did not induce tolerance in our studies'.

Instead of paying attention to this, science reporters – and many immunologists – concentrated on the results reported by Debbie Lenschow at the University of Chicago. She had induced tolerance in her experiments with CTLA4Ig. It was widely assumed that she had done something right that Linsley and his colleagues had done wrong.

Linsley himself couldn't account for the discrepancy. But he doubted that tolerance, in the sense that other immunologists intended, was a valid concept. He wasn't sure there was a simple switch you could just flip to create permanent tolerance to a specific foreign antigen. He wasn't sure that there had been anything 'permanent' about Lenschow's results – or Medawar's for that matter.

In the wake of the two CTLA4Ig papers in *Science*, Linsley was invited to a series of conferences on the topic. One of these was convened at NIH in Bethesda, Maryland. It was a big gathering, to which everyone who was anyone in transplant and theoretical immunology had been invited. About seventy men and women sat around an enormous table. Linsley arrived, sat down at his place, and listened as a fellow scientist, the conference convener, opened by saying: perhaps we could go around the table and have each person tell us what he means by tolerance.

As Linsley expected, there were some major conceptual divisions. The voicing of all these different opinions took about an hour. The theoretical immunologists, such as Marc Jenkins, spoke of permanent transformation of nonself antigens into 'self', from the point of view of the immune system. Others weren't sure that was possible, or necessary. The transplant surgeons sitting around the table didn't even seem to care about 'tolerance'. All they cared about was keeping transplant patients alive and healthy with minimum immunosuppression. If it took six months of daily doses with CTLA4Ig to make a transplanted organ 'take', and if CTLA4Ig was less toxic than cyclosporine, then that would be wonderful. It would be a big advance for them – a huge step beyond cyclosporine.

Already Linsley was doubtful that CTLA4Ig could do even that. The drug worked wonderfully in rodents, but even in rodents, as Linsley had found, it didn't usually induce permanent tolerance, and it sometimes failed to do its primary job of preventing transplant rejection.

Experiments in monkeys, whose immune systems were much more like human immune systems, would be still more sobering. In the five years following the first Linsley and Lenschow experiments with rodents, no one would be able to prevent organ transplant rejection in monkeys using CTLA4Ig. Jeff Bluestone's lab would try, but would fail; after that only one other lab even attempted it. Monkey experiments were enormously expensive. The best that seemed possible was that rejection in monkeys could be moderately delayed with CTLA4Ig, but not prevented. In humans, as everyone knew, the results would certainly be no better.

Even if it was used as an adjunct to conventional therapies such as cyclosporine, CTLA4Ig would have to perform a difficult, inhibitory function – blocking all proteins of a certain type (B7) to prevent their activity, instead of merely binding, like an activity-stimulating hormone, to a sensitive few. That meant that CTLA4Ig would have to be used in very high doses. And no one yet knew how to put it in pill form – so it would have to be delivered intravenously, inside a hospital room. All of which meant that it would be very expensive, perhaps prohibitively expensive. Genentech and Biogen, who had been developing CD4Ig drugs to block HIV, had abandoned those drugs for similar reasons. They worked well in the test tube, and even in rodents. But in the human body – in the real world of medicine – they did too little to be effective.

The years went by and CTLA4Ig, despite the sensation it had caused in 1992, never regained the headlines. Bristol Myers Squibb eventually set up clinical trials of the drug in humans – but in patients with severe psoriasis. Patients with severe psoriasis were not a 10 billion dollar market. They were the people through whom Bristol Myers Squibb saved face, a little. By late 1997 it was clear that CTLA4Ig had some effectiveness for these patients. But only some. That year BMS closed down its Seattle branch. Peter Linsley and Jeff Ledbetter joined other biotech firms in Seattle, and started to work in unrelated areas of research.

The Grail, once again, had vanished into the mists.

14

Twelve Monkeys

'Things don't work. They go wrong. Animals die.'

For David Harlan, in the days before things suddenly began to go right, there were only the deaths of monkey to contemplate: deaths due to the failure of CTLA4Ig. And it reminded Harlan why he disliked medical research – why he had once, in fact, decided not to be a medical researcher.

As a senior pre-med student at the University of Michigan, Harlan had worked in a laboratory, a few hours a day. The research had to do with the regulation of cardiovascular blood flow, and the research subjects were dogs. Often Harlan would visit the room where the dogs lay in their cages and he would see that one of the dogs, despite all Harlan's efforts, all the neuralgic tedium of laboratory methods, had unexpectedly died, probably in agony. At other times a dog lived to the end of an experiment only to be sacrificed, as the doctors called it, its body opened and its arteries studied. Harlan would always remember how the dogs licked his face or his hands, in simple canine offerings of affection, while he concentrated on administering the intravenous solution that would kill them.

Harlan did not do further research until, with six months free before he started an internship at Duke University Medical Center, he reluctantly took another job in a laboratory. He needed the money. But again it was cardiovascular research, and again the research was inflicted upon dogs. And again the dogs licked his face and hands when the experiments ended and it was time for him to hold them still as he quietly filled their bloodstreams with deadly doses of penthothal.

Harlan avoided research and instead became a doctor. He did his internship and his residency at Duke and during his second year of

residency he was voted best house doctor by his peers. He looked
in those days, as now, somewhat like Doctor Green in the TV series
ER, though his face was thinner and his glasses squarer, and he had
a fuller head of hair, cut short to Navy regulations. The US Navy had
paid Harlan's medical school bills and he owed them time. He spent
four years at a navy hospital in San Diego, teaching and practising
internal medicine. He loved those years; he would say later that they
were probably the best in his life.

Harlan was enticed back to science for the usual reason: the recognition that mere doctors, increasingly, are only as good as the tools
scientists give them.

He ended up, in the early 1990s, in a laboratory at the Navy
Medical Research Institute, run by an oncologist and transplant
immunologist named Carl June. Now a navy captain, June was about
to retire and rejoin the lab as a civilian contractor. He also was about
to face the horror of his wife's battle with cancer.* Coincidentally,
he had become interested in studying how B7 receptors, rather than
being blocked by drugs, could instead be 'upregulated' on cancer cells
– made to sprout more profusely – so T cells could recognize and kill
those cancerous cells more easily. June wanted Harlan to work on
the other side of the lab, the side concerned with downregulating
B7/CD28 signalling, to cure transplant rejection and autoimmune
disease and other problems caused by marauding T cells.

Shortly after Harlan had joined the lab, news broke about Peter
Linsley's CTLA4Ig, the strange molecule that blocked B7 so well,
and Harlan decided to concentrate on that. He set up mouse transplant models and started using CTLA4Ig and anti–B7 antibodies to
prevent transplant rejection. Eventually, he decided to test the drug
in monkeys.

Harlan needed a transplant surgeon to carry out the experiments.
He searched for one, for a few months, and got nowhere. Then one

---

* Mrs June survived her ordeal, which involved lethal doses of chemotherapy, not
radiation, and an 'autologous' transplant of her own bone marrow that had been
harvested before she began receiving chemo. Because the marrow was her own (the
cancer was in her ovaries, not her blood cells) there was no risk of the GVHD that
had killed Maria Morderas and thousands of other 'allogeneic' (other-gened) marrow
transplant recipients.

day a Navy lieutenant commander named Allan Kirk walked into his office. Fresh-faced, farmboyish, thirty-one years old and with a brand-new immunology PhD to go with his Duke University MD, Kirk had just been accepted to the University of Wisconsin on a fellowship to study transplant surgery. The Navy didn't want him to study transplant surgery, however. The Navy had once been interested in transplant surgery – back in the days when Carl June and Craig Thompson had been sent out to Seattle – but those days were over; the programme had been transferred to the Army. What the Navy wanted now were regular all-round doctors who would go to sea on ships and subs, would man hospitals at shore bases.

Nevertheless, Kirk had his heart set on transplant surgery and he wanted Harlan's lab to sponsor him. Kirk was the kind of man who could slack sails and change tack with jaw-dropping suddenness, but he didn't like anyone else to set his course. He had once been a professional tuba player, if you can believe that. He had played tuba with the Virginia Philharmonic and was up in Boston one night, about to spend a year with the Boston Symphony, about to sign the lease for an apartment, and his fiancée was beside him, the girl he'd dated since elementary school, and everything was set and he was already, at nineteen, a successful musician – and just then, out of the blue, he decided he wanted to be a transplant surgeon.

Years later he couldn't really explain it. Perhaps it had been inside him, brewing, for a long time. In any case he knew now he wanted to be a transplant surgeon. Right out on the edge of medicine. He set that course and let nothing get in his way. He spent two years taking pre-med classes down at Old Dominion University, where his father was a botany professor and dean of the sciences, and he earned straight As and went to Duke, one of the premier med schools in the country. Duke was also one of the most expensive, which was why Kirk got the Navy to pay his way. But the Navy was never able to shackle him to a ship. A few months after he met Dave Harlan, he was up in Wisconsin starting his transplant surgery fellowship, and setting up an experiment to test CTLA4Ig in monkeys.

The transplant programme at the University of Wisconsin was run by a surgeon named Hans Sollinger. One of his young colleagues, Stuart Knechtle, had been a resident with Kirk down at Duke

and had invited Kirk up to study transplant surgery. Knechtle
had recently made use of a large primate centre at the university
to develop a new kidney transplant model in rhesus macaques.
Macaques are about as close to being human, immunologically, as
one can get in the animal world. And because they are so small they
don't require much of whatever protein or compound is being tested.
They are often the last stop for a new drug before it goes into homo
sapiens.

Essentially the Knechtle model was a tried-and-true set of surgical
procedures for extracting both kidneys from one rhesus macaque
monkey and replacing them with one kidney from a genetically
mismatched macaque donor. Without treatment, the monkey who
received such a mismatched transplant would quickly die, as his T
cells attacked the donated kidney and his kidney function went to
zero. The point was to test new transplant rejection drugs in the
monkeys, to keep them and their kidneys from dying. Dave Harlan,
remembering all the dogs he had had to kill in days past, was glad
he wasn't the one getting his hands bloody in this.

In the next year and a half Allan Kirk would run experiments
on twelve monkeys. These were monkeys that had come either
from the primate centre at the university or from a commercial
breeding colony down in Yemasee, South Carolina. Their fathers
and mothers were wild macaques who had swung and screeched
and gulped bananas in the jungles of Asia until the day that some
cigarette-smoking Indian or Malaysian or Vietnamese or Filipino had
enticed them into traps and roughly hauled them away. There had
been a major scare over Ebola virus in 1990 – many of the imported
Asian monkeys carried it in their blood – and though it appeared that
Asian Ebola posed no threat to humans it could certainly wreak havoc
among captive monkeys. So the importation of monkeys for research
had been cut down almost to nothing.

The monkeys were bred instead in large zoo-like colonies scattered
around the USA, and they were expensive. Each one cost $3,000, but
that was just the start. A monkey in a transplant experiment also had
to be housed and fed, and medically tested in half a dozen ways,
and injected with antibiotics and painkillers, and operated on, and
monitored, and autopsied – and it all added up to about $20,000 per
monkey.

   The Navy and Hans Sollinger's transplant surgery department, thankfully, were willing to take care of that expense. So Dave Harlan arranged with Genetics Institute for some precious ampules of CTLA4Ig, and sent them up to Kirk in Wisconsin, and Kirk and Stuart Knechtle started experimenting.

   Knechtle had been running his own series of monkey transplants, testing a new anti-rejection drug called CRM19*. Every month or so, when he had a day free from doing human transplant surgery, Knechtle – assisted by various nurses and helpers and other young transplant surgeons, including Kirk – would have two monkeys brought into the veterinary operating room for one of the experimental transplants. Knechtle agreed to work two additional monkeys into the rotation for Kirk; they would be given CTLA4Ig as an anti-rejection drug, instead of CRM19.

The veterinary operating room sat in a wing at one end of the university medical centre, adjacent to the animal pens. On the morning of the first CTLA4Ig experiment two macaques were wheeled in, limp and glazed with shots of ketamine. They were adolescent males, about two years old, thin brownish-grey, hairy-faced boy monkeys. The kind of monkeys that used to sit on the shoulders of pirates and organ-grinders. They were about twelve inches long head to toe, and weighed six pounds. Next to all the masked and gowned humans, all the bald, big-headed, deep-voiced higher primates, they looked very small and fragile.

   When everything was ready an anaesthetist put tubes into the monkey's noses, down their windpipes, feeding their tiny lungs a solution of air mixed with halothane sleep gas. Knechtle and Kirk each opened up one monkey. The donor had two kidneys, and one was cut out and placed in a tray with a saline solution. The recipient had already donated one of his kidneys a month before, as part of Knechtle's experimental series. His last kidney now was taken out – and thrown away – and the kidney taken from the donor was sewn in.

   When all the right vessels had been hooked up or tied off both

---

* CRMI9 is an immunotoxin – a congugate of an antibody specific for the T-cell CD3 receptor, and a cell-killing protein known as diptheria toxin. It effectively wipes out the T-cell population for a period of a few weeks.

monkeys were sutured closed again. They received aspirin and a shot of butorphanol for pain, and trimethoprim–sulfa against bacterial infection from the surgery.

The monkey who had received a donated kidney was also given a shot of 30 milligrams of CTLA4Ig. Then he and the other monkey were taken to their small concrete-floored holding room, down the hall, and put – still asleep – in separate cages. An electric heater was placed in the room, and each monkey was wrapped in a blanket. Little monkeys lost heat quickly when they were inactive.

Other monkeys, survivors of Knechtle's experiments, were in the surrounding cages. They eyed the newcomers, perhaps wondering: who among us will be luckiest – and die quickly?

Every eight hours, for the next day or so, Kirk and one of the Knechtle lab anaesthesiologists visited the monkeys. The two men quieted the macaques with ketamine, gave them shots of trimethoprim and painkilling butorphanol, gave them IV boluses of nutrient-filled fluid.

On day one – the day after the transplant – the monkey who had received the mismatched kidney was given his second 30 milligram shot of CTLA4Ig. On day two he was given yet another shot of CTLA4Ig, and this time, instead of being fed intravenously, he began to eat solid food. On day seven his surgical sutures were removed.

Occasionally in his series of transplants designed to test CRM19 Stuart Knechtle put a mismatched kidney into a monkey and gave him no anti-rejection treatment at all. The monkey – eventually there would be four of these controls, shared between Knechtle's and Kirk's experiments – started downhill right away. As his enraged T cells infiltrated and swelled and began to destroy his new kidney, his bloodstream level of creatinine, a key measure of kidney function, flew up and out of the normal range. Waste metabolites that should have been passed out of the body through the kidney instead built up in his blood. The monkey grew lethargic, stopped passing urine, and when it was obvious that the end was near he was put to death mercifully with a large injection of sodium pentothal plus potassium chloride. In the four control monkeys this quiet end came on day 5, 7, 7, and 8 after transplant. That is to say, the end came quickly for all of them.

But the first monkey to receive CTLA4Ig lasted longer than that. His course of CTLA4Ig, at 30 milligrams per day, ended after five days but he remained healthy on day 6. Another week went by and still he seemed healthy.

Each monkey had been tattooed, not long after birth, with an identification code on his chest or leg. This first monkey had been tattooed with the code 1GD. Allan Kirk liked to associate these abstract codes with real words. But nothing sprung to mind for 1GD, until around day 17 when 1GD showed unmistakable signs of decline. His creatinine levels were suddenly sky-high. The GD now meant 'God Damn'. On day 20 Kirk saw the monkey lying motionless in his cage and knew it was time to put him down. A lab assistant held him, and Kirk injected him with the pentothal solution, and the monkey went limp and within a few minutes stopped breathing. The lab assistant carried him to the animal pathology room, where an autopsy was done to verify that the donated kidney had been rejected.

The monkey who had donated his kidney to 1GD was tattooed with the label EK. The same initials, thought Kirk, as his son Eric. A few weeks after the death of 1GD, little EK had his remaining kidney removed and replaced with a kidney that belonged to yet another monkey who lay on an operating table several feet away. EK was given 60 milligrams of CTLA4Ig on day zero, the day of surgery – a massive dose for an animal his size, twice what 1GD had been given – then 30 milligrams on days 2, 4, 6, 8, 10, and 12. He lived longer than 1GD had lived. He passed day 20 and kept going, doing fine though he had not been given CTLA4Ig for a week. He was floating without a parachute.

Every day Allan Kirk tried to steal a few minutes from the rest of his schedule to visit little EK. Kirk was working full-time as a transplant surgeon for human patients, and while there were slow days when patients neared death awaiting organs that weren't available there also were insane, fatigue-blurred days when two, three donated organs suddenly arrived in little plastic coolers, all at once, carried by air couriers and helicopter, and it was all hands on deck until the patients could be wheeled into the operating room on gurneys, one by one, and the new organs put in and stabilized, the stack of organ coolers in the operating room growing shorter and shorter until there was nothing left to transplant and Kirk squinted at the clock and saw that an entire day, perhaps a day and half, had passed.

On day 28 for little monkey EK, Kirk walked into the monkey room and saw that EK seemed less active. A creatinine test showed why. The creatinine level had spiked. His kidney, suddenly under attack from T cells, had almost stopped working. Two days later, on day 30, Kirk had to put EK down. He didn't want to think about EK's nickname any more. Once again a lab assistant carried the little curled ball of monkey fur down to the autopsy room.

Two dead monkeys, and nothing to show for them.

By this time Allan Kirk, and Dave Harlan back in Maryland, had heard that Jeff Bluestone's lab in Chicago also had tried CTLA4Ig in macaques. Bluestone's people had tried using CTLA4Ig to prevent the rejection of insulin cell transplants. The CTLA4Ig had failed there, too, though Kirk and Harlan, like many other transplant immunologists, considered insulin cell transplants too messy, too fraught with problems, to use as a testbed for CTLA4Ig. If the transplant didn't take, you didn't know if it was because the drug had failed to work. It might have been some other problem. The Knechtle kidney transplant model, by contrast, seemed to amount to a much more robust test. If a transplant didn't take, in the Knechtle model, it was almost certainly because the anti-rejection drug had failed to work. The Knechtle model, in other words, was the most definitive test available. And CTLA4Ig had failed it. Which meant that CTLA4Ig was dead, as a transplant-rejection drug that would usher in some new age of medicine. It couldn't even beat old cyclosporine.

The wheel of discovery and enthusiasm had now turned full circle, it seemed, yet had not really taken scientists anywhere. Carl June and Jeff Ledbetter and Craig Thompson and Jeff Bluestone and everybody else who had been working on the problem were ten years older. But they faced the same problem they had faced with cyclosporine. Cyclosporine blocked one T-cell activation pathway, but it couldn't stop transplant rejection. Faced with that, the immunologists had gone out and discovered a second T-cell activation pathway, and had figured out a way to block that one – had even figured out, they thought, how to use that second pathway to induce 'tolerance' to specific antigens. But still, when they put the theory into action in human-like immune systems, in those now-dead monkeys, it had failed to work.

What was wrong? Was there yet another T-cell activation pathway out there? A *third* pathway that everyone had missed?

One spring day in 1996 Dave Harlan attended a conference organized by the US military's Uniformed Health Sciences University. The conference was being held on his own campus, there at the Navy Medical Center in Bethesda, just a short walk from his office. At the conference Harlan listened as a scientist named Chris Larsen from Emory University in Atlanta read a paper about a transplant experiment he and a team had recently performed. It was another mouse experiment.

Each mouse in the experiment had received a mismatched heart, plus mismatched skin grafts, and Larsen had used a two-drug combination to make the transplants take. Harlan, hearing that, was moderately impressed. Heart transplants were hard to do properly under the best circumstances. And mismatched skin was more resistant to successful transplantation than almost any other piece of tissue. A foreign skin cell, to an angry T cell, was like the proverbial red rag to a bull.

Larsen and his group had made the transplants take by giving the mice CTLA4Ig plus another new drug called MR1, a monoclonal antibody. MR1 bound to a T-cell receptor that didn't even have a name yet. Everyone was calling this T-cell receptor CD40 ligand, or CD40L, because it normally bound to a receptor called CD40.

Not much was known about CD40 either. If you looked back through the literature, you would find almost nothing published on it before 1993. But apparently it sprouted from the surfaces of antigen-presenting cells, and apparently it interacted with some ligand – CD40L – on T cells. Either CD40 was a signalling device antigen-presenting cells used to kick T cells to do their part, or CD40L was a signalling device T cells used to kick antigen-presenting cells to do their part. Or both. No one was sure.

Still, the CD40/CD40L pathway did seem fairly important. A paper published in *Nature* in 1995, by researchers at Yale led by Iqbal Grewal, told of the genetic engineering of mouse T cells that did not express CD40L. That was always a good way to find out what a protein did: remove it, and see what happened as a result.

What happened in the case of the CD40L-deficient mouse T cells was that they were unable to go into full battle mode when presented with antigens under ordinary, *in vivo* conditions. You could prick these mice with a variety of antigens – keyhole limpet hemocyanin and cytochrome c, to name two – and their T cells would not get angry, would not proliferate into populous clones specific for those antigens. Their T cells had more or less been neutered. And so had their B cells: these mice couldn't make proper antibody responses to disease.

There were humans, too, who suffered from a condition like this. They had a genetic flaw that prevented CD40L from being expressed on their T cells, and perhaps as a result (there is still debate over this) they suffered from a condition akin to Aids. They succumbed to opportunistic infections such as *P. carinii* pneumonia and *cryptosporidium* diarrhoea. Until 1993 no one knew what their underlying problem was. Then CD40 and CD40L were cloned and sequenced, and scientists began to understand what might be going wrong.

It sounded like good news, finding another immune-cell activation pathway. But – what a chaos! It was dismayingly evident now that the society of immune cells seethed with complexity, with secret handshakes and deals, with coded messages whispered across crowded, smoke-filled rooms.

Yet the bottom line for transplant work might still be simple: if you could block the CD40/CD40L pathway, perhaps only for a few days or weeks, you would probably have much better luck with whatever other anti-rejection drugs you were using.

That is what Chris Larsen and his group tried, when they transplanted hearts and skin from mouse to mismatched mouse. They used CTLA4Ig because the evidence suggested that it would help. They also used MR1, because MR1 blocked CD40L.

Some of the mice got one drug or the other, and others got both. Most of them died, either from heart-transplant-rejection or because they were 'sacrificed' two months after transplant. But there was something very hopeful about what had happened to them.

Those mice that had received only one of the two drugs – or, say, CTLA4Ig plus cyclosporine – showed evidence, at autopsy, that the immune system had started to reject the transplanted organs. Those that had received both CTLA4Ig and MR1, by contrast, looked as if their new hearts, and new patches of skin, had always been theirs. Speaking of the skin grafts Larsen exulted: 'Fifty days after transplantation these allografts remained healthy in appearance, well vascularized, supple, and bearing short white hair.' Hallelujah!

After listening to Larsen's talk, Harlan asked him a few questions, then walked back to his office. He was already planning his next experiment with the monkeys up in Wisconsin.

MR1, the monoclonal antibody that bound to CD40L, was just a test reagent made in a lab at Dartmouth University run by immunologist Randy Noelle. Peter Linsley's lab at Bristol Myers Squibb had picked up commercial rights, but MRI had been made only for mouse CD40L. It might not work as well against the CD40L proteins on the cells of monkeys and humans. On the other hand, Biogen Co., up in Boston, had a human-ish anti-CD40L monoclonal antibody, and a strong patent on it. No competitor could touch Biogen when it came to the CD40 pathway. Biogen's monoclonal had the romantic, evocative name 5C8.

Harlan went to his phone, arranged to get some 5C8 from Biogen, and some more CTLA4Ig from Genetics Institute. In a few months all the paperwork had been signed and the drugs were in the hands of Allan Kirk.

In Madison, Wisconsin, it was now August 1996. Kirk, raised in Virginia and North Carolina, and still with bit of that aw-shucks old-swamp molasses in his voice, had already endured one Nearctic winter here, and was weeks away from being subjected to another. The buildings on the university campus were mostly connected by closed, heatable walkways, as if this were a lonely outpost on some inhumanly cold planet. Wisconsin could be like that. But the snow hadn't started yet and the flowers were still in bloom. The sap was still high. Kirk went to the university animal pens one day and selected eight monkeys. Perhaps they would not all die this time.

The first monkey to receive the combined drugs was tattooed with the number 1295, a label hard to turn into a nickname. He got a whopping dose of 60 milligrams of each drug. Kirk injected him with the first doses at the time of the operation, then every other day up to day 16. The monkey lay for each injection on the examination table across from the cages, dopey with ketamine, cradled by a lab assistant. Around day 28, the time point when EK's kidney had begun to show signs of rejection, 1295 also started to show the signs. He was put to death on day 32. It seemed that the combination of the drugs had made no difference at all.

As 1295 lay dying in the monkey room, one of the other macaques watched him with what might have been special interest. This monkey, RQ1336, had donated one of his kidneys to 1295. That kidney, that piece of him, was dying inside of 1295. And now the surgeons in their blue smocks had taken RQ1336's remaining kidney out, and had put a new one in, from some other monkey. And had started him on the same dosing schedule with the two drugs. He might have wondered whether he was witnessing, in the death spasms of 1295, his own near-future.

But RQ1336 sailed through the rejection barrier that seemed to hit the other animals around day 28. And he kept going – five weeks, six weeks, seven weeks, eight weeks. Kirk, finishing a kidney transplant operation late at night, would shower and change his scrubs and walk down to the monkey room, just to see how little RQ1336 was doing. RQ1336! He was like Ham, that chimp that NASA had fired successfully into space before risking any of the Mercury astronauts' hides. But in RQ1336's case, there was no telling when his ship would come down. He kept speeding past milestones: nine weeks, ten weeks, eleven weeks. He was cruising. He played around in his cage with his cagemate, a macaque from one of Knechtle's experiments. He looked healthy. His creatinine levels were fine, perfectly normal. Twelve weeks, thirteen weeks. Fourteen weeks! The monkey, following only eight doses of anti-rejection drugs, had not had any anti-rejection therapy for nearly three months now. Nothing like that had ever been achieved in a primate. There seemed to be no harmful side-effects at all. Whatever other antigens RQ1336 had become tolerized to, during that eight-day course of therapy, they apparently had not been dangerous ones. He did not suffer opportunistic infections. He was not sprouting with cancers. He seemed the very picture of a healthy, happy monkey.

At day 100 Kirk gave RQ1336 a blood test and found that

his creatinine level had suddenly doubled. His kidney was now under attack. If past experience was anything to go by, he would be dead, his kidney a wasteland of T-cell-killed tissue, within another week.

Kirk decided to try to save little RQ1336, with a second sixteen-day course of the two drugs. And he did. After just a few days with the resumed dosages of the drugs, the monkey's creatinine levels went back down to baseline. Lab tests showed that the animal's T cells had lost reactivity to antigens from the donor monkey – even though they had not lost reactivity to other antigens. That was good. It meant that the monkey was tolerating his new kidney, but still had the rest of his immune system intact. That was the dream. And RQ1336 kept going.

Around day 150 several of the macaques in the monkey room, including untreated ones, became sick with enterocolitis. RQ1336 began to lose weight. The protocol in such trials specified that, for mercy's sake, for the sake of ethics, when a monkey had lost fifteen per cent of its baseline weight it should be put down. On day 165 the pioneering transplant survivor fell below that line, and Allan Kirk and an assistant were obliged to go in and euthanize him with pentothal. In the autopsy room they found that he had indeed been sick because of the enterocolitis, caused by a kind of bacterium called campylobacter. His transplanted kidney was fine.

Two other monkeys, watching the death of RQ1336 from their cages, had received new kidneys days apart from each other. They had gone through a day 0 to day 16 regimen of the two drugs, with an extra dose at day 28 to boost them past the rejection monster that seemed to lie in wait out there. On the day that RQ1336 died, they were at day 90 and 96, respectively. They had not had any rejection episodes. Their creatinine levels seemed to be pegged to baseline. They appeared able to ward off colds and flu and cancers as well as any other monkeys. They appeared to be normal except for the fact that each was missing a kidney and had a surgical scar to show for it.

The two monkeys, 2HP and DJD, are still alive as I write, almost a year after they received their transplants and their short courses of CTLA4Ig and 5C8.

Two other monkeys in the experiment, BPV and DEA, received not two drugs but one: 5C8 alone, every other day from day 0 to day 16 after transplant. To Allan Kirk's and everyone else's surprise, both monkeys made it easily to three months without a rejection episode. Their kidneys started to come under T–cell attack around day 90, but both recovered quickly with an extra seven doses of 5C8. So there were two monsters out there, at one month and three months, but they both could be beaten.*

About seven months after these monkeys had been transplanted, one of them, DEA, was given a skin graft from the same monkey whose kidney he now had working inside him. Kirk knew that skin grafts were the toughest things to transplant, but he was going for all the marbles. If he could get a skin transplant from the same mismatched donor to take, without additional dosing of an anti-rejection drug – well, that would be it: that would be the Grail of transplant immunology. True and complete tolerance to donor-specific tissue. Tolerance even to transplanted skin! Just like Peter Medawar's old experiment, but now in adolescent monkeys, just one small step from men. If he could make this one work, Kirk could go home and dust off a space on his mantel for the little Nobel Prize medal, in its attractive holder, that would surely be sitting there some day.

But when the dust had cleared from this experiment Allan Kirk would react to the word tolerance as if it were bad luck.

The grafted skin lasted on the back of DEA for two months, which was amazing in itself. For those two months Allan Kirk, and back in Maryland Dave Harlan and Carl June, were walking on air. That was when I first spoke to them. They had already accomplished something no other immunologist had accomplished, something that every other immunologist wanted to accomplish, and it seemed that they were about to go even further.

---

* The last two monkeys in the Wisconsin series, CET and DCP, received the same total amount of 5C8, but were dosed over 28 days instead of 16. One, DCP, had a rejection episode at day 110, more or less like BPV and DEA. The other, CET, had no rejection episodes and, at the time of writing, remains hale and hearty more than a year and a half after receiving his last dose of 5C8. Harland and Kirk have since treated four more monkeys at a Navy facility near their lab in Bethesda. With the same 28-day dosing regimen, none has had a rejection episode in the six months since their last doses of 5C8.

But slowly, around day 60 following the graft, the piece of donor skin on the back of monkey DEA started to turn pink. A host of T cells, armed against the donor antigens but sedated for eight months by the two short courses of 5C8, had been gradually roused again by the invasion of the irksome skin tissue. And as they attacked the skin, and their battle cries and chemical fumes swirled around the body, the T cells noticed the kidney that also seemed foreign, also belonged to the invader. And the kidney came under attack, too.

Kirk could have retreated the monkey with 5C8, to stop the rejection of the donor kidney that had already lasted so long, but he and Knechtle and Dave Harlan had agreed in advance not to. The idea was to see if such episodes could resolve on their own. This one didn't. Nine months after he had received his mismatched kidney, monkey DEA succumbed to renal failure brought about by immune rejection. With him died, perhaps for ever, the dream of true tolerance, the myth of the immunological Holy Grail.

15

We Can All Go Home Now

But – so what if the Holy Grail was just a myth? So what if 'permanent donor-specific tolerance' was not yet achievable – or perhaps not even possible? Allan Kirk and Dave Harlan, and the other immunologists on whose shoulders they stood, had achieved something virtually as good: prolonged survival of mismatched transplants, evidently maintainable with occasional short courses of 5C8 alone.

The fact that that skin graft had lasted two months, in the absence of any immunosuppression or anti-rejection therapy, suggested that transplant technology had taken a giant leap forward. Remember also that the transplanted kidneys were highly mismatched. They were about as different, in their MHC make-up, as one could get within the same species. To make such transplants take, with previous-generation drugs like cyclosporine, usually meant years of toxic immunosuppression, and huge risks of opportunistic infections and cancers. But if the monkey results held up, all that would disappear. The dark ages of transplant technology would now start to slip back into history, like smallpox and plague and scurvy.

Allan Kirk, wearing his Navy service-dress blue uniform, gave a lecture announcing preliminary results of the monkey experiment at the annual meeting of the American Society of Transplant Surgeons, in a darkened conference room in a hotel in Chicago in early May 1997. Dave Harlan, also in uniform, was in the audience. The audience, most of them surgeons at big teaching hospitals, must have wondered what these Navy officers were doing. The Navy? Who ever heard of a medical advance coming from the Navy? Or from anywhere in the military. All too often, military surgeons were surgeons who couldn't make it in the real world.

The applause at the end of Kirk's address was polite, but definitely not overwhelming.

Still, there was a small buzz of interest. Harlan stood with Kirk afterwards and several surgeons came up to offer congratulations. One of them was Ron Shapiro, head of kidney transplant surgery at the University of Pittsburgh. He looked at the two Navy officers, then said with an air of genial puzzlement: 'Did I misunderstand you, or did you just say you've got the answer – and we can all go home now?'

The conference made no impact on the rest of the world. There was no mention of Kirk and Harlan's monkey transplants in the media. The stock price of Biogen, which stood to gain enormously from the success of 5C8, remained near its fifty-two-week low. Biogen shares even dipped for a while after an analyst on Wall Street, apparently unaware of the 5C8 work, noted dourly that the company had no blockbuster drugs coming through its production pipeline, and was overvalued. Science journalists, who relied largely on press releases for news of what was happening on their beat, received no such press release, and therefore knew nothing.

That would change, however. NMRI, having gone to the trouble of supporting a scientific research facility, and funding the expensive transplant experiments in monkeys (why must medical science be funded by a war-fighting agency? a budget-minded congressman might have asked), wanted to show off what it had accomplished. After Kirk and Harlan's paper on the experiments was accepted by *Proceedings of the National Academy of Sciences*, and a publication date of 5 August was set, the creaky NMRI publicity machine was wheeled into position. Harlan and Kirk were forbidden to speak to journalists until the appointed day – when the press releases were faxed out and a news conference was held in the Pentagon, and Kirk and Harlan were surrounded by gleaming brass, everybody in dress-whites. The assembled journalists were not science correspondents, however; they were Pentagon correspondents. That was how these things had to be done. But the Pentagon correspondents passed on their notes to science correspondents, and TV trucks began arriving on the grassy campus of the Navy Medical Center, just across Rockville Pike from NIH, and Kirk and Harlan talked and talked, for the print media and radio reporters and TV reporters, and the next day they were flown to the Manhattan studio of *Good Morning America*, and were introduced to the world – two young, clean–cut, handsome and gentlemanly officers in their navy dress–whites – as the fellows who had developed the answer to transplants. It was hard even to begin to get across the complex reality of transplant immunology, in the couple of minutes available to them. They might as well have been talking about the physics of black holes. But it was clear that transplanting mismatched organs was a good possibility now. And the host thanked them and – hey, keep up the good work, fellas, and . . . now, our next guest—

Soon the public interest subsided to a trickle of e–mails and phone calls. One man telephoned to know if the navy doctors could give his dog a heart transplant. A woman dissatisfied with her eyebrows inquired about the possibility of an eyebrow transplant.

But if the public didn't fully grasp the consequences of what had just happened, up in Wisconsin, the network of transplant surgeons and scientists certainly did. Theorists scrambled to figure out the implications of the Wisconsin data. How did 5C8 work? Probably most compellingly, immunologist Polly Matzinger and colleagues proposed that it worked by blocking a key handshake in a three–way interaction between T cells and antigen–presenting cells (APCs). In this new 'license to kill' model, a 'helper' T cell that encounters an APC bearing the right antigen locks its CD40L receptors onto the APC's CD40 receptors. This coupling switches the APC into battle mode: it now can license 'killer' T cells it encounters to go out and destroy any cells it finds bearing those antigens. If the CD40L/CD40 link is blocked for a time by 5C8 or some such agent, APCs fail to go into battle mode, and therefore can't license killer T cells to kill.

In the context of organ transplants, a month or two of 5C8 doses would essentially prevent killer T cells from doing significant damage (perhaps even switching the killer T cells specific for donor antigens into a short–lived anergy or 'off mode') during the most critical period when a new organ slowly becomes integrated into its host body and is otherwise relatively exposed to the storms of the immune system.

Why 5C8 should work so much better, in this sense, than CTLA4Ig and cyclosporine – the blockers of two other T cell activation pathways – no one knew for certain. But by the time I put this book to bed, Biogen was already setting up human clinical trials of the drug in several applications, ranging from a rare autoimmune disease known as idiopathic thrombocytopenic purpura to kidney transplants and even islet cell transplants – which with previous drugs have not really been successful in humans – to cure juvenile diabetes. New experimental transplant centers were being set up at Harvard, NIH, and the University of Washington in Seattle to take rapid advantage of 5C8 and other new anti-rejection drugs.

The first human trials of 5C8 to prevent transplant rejection will probably take place in late 1998, and if all goes well, the drug will enter regular clinical use some time in the first few years of the new millennium.

16

The Selfish Self

Some day old age will be a dream from which we wake.

'How do you feel?' the nurse asks as I stir in the bed.

'Ah, uh, fee—' I feel different. My voice doesn't work as it should. My muscles are nearly paralysed. The room moves around me slightly and I can make only a little sense of what I see. Walls, a large TV screen, the nurse, my wife (my seventh?), another older-looking woman. My thoughts are a jumble. A fraction of my life, my self, which is to say my brain, has been burned away – a bit here, a bit there – to make room for new stuff, for fresh, lab-grown baby neurons with which my cranium has been pumped full. My cranium – actually my old cranium is gone. What was inside it has been plopped into, rewired to, a new body that looks, and despite the temporary paralysis already vaguely feels, like a younger version of me. Except that it is, genetically and synthetically, a good deal better than a younger version of me. And the rewiring isn't quite finished; for that the brain and body need experience. It will be a month before we, brain and body, can talk or see or move properly. Three months before we can run. Already we – I – have a nagging sense that there are blank places where memories used to be, where green paths run suddenly into dark, formless dead-ends. What was I before? Who am I now? I am someone else, though there is a core of me that is still me.

Genes were once the only biological entities that could be immortal. They ran and fought their way through history, everlasting shapeshifters shedding bodies every generation, sexually mixing themselves, forming new bodies, dying out, mutating their way back into existence, spreading themselves around as well as they could. Selfish genes and selfish gangs of genes. But now has come the age of the selfish self, the self that sheds genes and everything else as it pleases, keeping immortal only its core of selfness, its consciousness that it is – through all those changes of environment – somehow the same beast that popped from its mother's bloody womb however many decades back.

'Wha – you –?' What do you think? I try to ask my wife, who is standing there by the bed. My wife had the operation – the Overhaul, people call it now – a year ago and became for a while a trophy wife, because she looked about twenty-two. Luckily she liked the idea of being married to a much older man. Then she started to tire me out. I knew it was time for me to get the Overhaul too.

'You look like a million bucks,' she says. With a twinkle in her ice-blue zoom-lens eyes – because she knows very well it cost more than that.

And the room blurs.

Because the future is blurry. Perhaps other, gentler technology will take over long before the Overhaul, the whole-body transplant, becomes a reality.

First things first. When transplants from human donors become easier, thanks to drugs like 5C8, it will push up the demand for transplantable organs. As I write, that demand is already soaring exponentially, while the supply has just about levelled off. In 1998 in America about 20,000 people will receive transplants, but three times that number – 60,000 – will languish on the waiting list, and of those about 5,000 will die waiting.

The availability of new anti-rejection drugs will only make that waiting list longer in the near-term, but less immediately, and less directly, it might also help to increase the supply of organs. As more people become eligible for organ transplants – because those transplants are easier and safer to perform successfully – their calls for greater organ donations will carry more and more weight with legislators. Only a small fraction of people now sign organ-donor agreements before they die. Perhaps the advent of good anti-rejection drugs will make it more obvious, to everyone, that laws should be passed making it easier – even automatic – for the organs of a newly-dead person to be harvested by doctors for transplant purposes.

Yet there are limits here. It is relatively uncommon for people to die in such a way that they are brain dead but their organs are healthy. The typical case is death by head injury in a traffic accident. Airbags, and better car designs, are keeping the number of those cases down – even as the demand for organs continues to rise sharply.

Another limit is a conceptual one. I think many younger people find it hard to agree to donate their organs because they find it hard to accept, deep down in their minds, that there will come a day when they won't need those organs. The logic of organ donation is one that young minds are not really designed to process. Trying to imagine one's own death, from the perspective of twenty or thirty or forty and rude health, is like trying to imagine the outside of the universe. It's better not to even think about it.

All of which means that people in search of spare parts, who don't want to stand in line for years, will soon have to find alternatives to parts harvested from dead people.

One much-talked-about possibility in this area goes by the name of xenotransplantation: the transplantation of tissue and organs from other species. You may have heard about transplants of baboon hearts into humans. Well, forget about that. Primates are too expensive for large-scale harvesting of organs, and probably too risky, in terms of disease transmission to humans. Pigs are what the transplant science community is talking about today. Pigs are cheap, and many of their organs are close enough to human to be functional. They also can be genetically engineered to make their cells even more 'human' – at which point, to ensure genetic quality control, they can even be cloned into farms of identical, generic, organ-providers. If you are a pig lover, this may sound a bit harsh. But consider: we already eat pigs – what can be worse than that?

There are still three major problems with transplanting pig organs into people. The first is that the kinds of organs a pig can provide are limited. Pig livers, pig kidneys, pig pancreases and pig hearts, should be fine for a human, but pig lungs, pig guts and pig skin might not be.

The second problem is that xenotransplants are inherently riskier than allotransplants (transplants from others within a species). The immune mechanisms at work are more powerful, and less well understood. If you were to put a pig heart into a human without any accompanying anti-rejection drugs it would be rejected not within days, as for an allotransplant, but within minutes. When xenotransplants occur a special antibody-and-complement attack mechanism switches on in the host body immediately, in a process called 'hyperacute rejection'.

Since 1995 various companies have claimed that they can genetically engineer pig cells to overcome the hyperacute rejection phase.
But that's not all there is to xenotransplant rejection. In the days
after the hyperacute rejection comes 'delayed xenograft rejection',
mediated by macrophages and natural killer cells; and after them
come the T cells. Experiments are underway in monkeys but it's
not yet clear that the current genetic engineering of pig cells, plus
sophisticated new drugs such as 5C8, will be able to overcome all
those modes of rejection.

Probably the most enduring problem for xenotransplants will be
the risk of transmitting diseases across species. The two worst disease
pandemics in developed countries this century started when viruses
jumped to homo sapiens from some other animal host. The flu virus
that killed 20 million people worldwide, in a few weeks in 1918, was
a genetic mix of human influenza virus and pig influenza virus. The
retrovirus HIV, which is arguably worse, is now thought to have
jumped from monkeys somewhere around 1940. And speaking of
retroviruses, strange new retroviruses have recently been found in
pigs genetically engineered for transplant work. These retroviruses
are able to infect and grow within human cells in lab cultures, and
they are also probably impossible to breed out of pigs, having inserted
themselves at multiple random points in pig genomes. Another hazard
to worry about here is the always-lethal 'prion' disease, or set of
diseases, that variously afflict humans (CJD, kuru), cattle (mad cow
disease), sheep (scrapie) and other species. What if such a thing got
loose in a clone of pigs on a transplant farm? How would we know –
before it was too late?

The disease risk from xenotransplants might prove more theoretical
than actual, but by the time we find out, we might have the technology
to leave pigs behind – to grow our own 'human' transplant organs in
the laboratory.

Jonathan Slack is a developmental biologist at the University of
Bath. His laboratory and the rest of the campus (an awful spawn
of 1960s modernist architecture, like something out of *A Clockwork
Orange*) is tucked out of sight on a hill above the relaxed Georgian
beauty of the old Roman outpost. Slack is the scientist behind that
news item you may have seen some time in the summer of 1997.
Scientists Take Step Toward Brave New World of Organ Farms.

Slack and his laboratory staff, by switching off certain key genes in the embryo of a species of frog, birthed a headless frog, a half-animal that – well, did nothing much besides exist. It had just enough frogness to be useful as a supplier of spare parts to other frogs, but not enough frogness that you would call it a real frog.

Naturally, people started to wonder: what if we did this to humans? And what if we combined the technique Slack used with the technology of cloning? What if we grew human clones to order – a headless clone for me, a headless clone for you – or, more cheaply and more realistically, grew generic human pieces for everyone, in bubbling tanks? Vast farms of human organs (livers on this ward, kidneys upstairs) to feed our voracious appetite for youth.

If it can be done in amphibians, how long will it take us to figure out how to do it in humans? I don't know. No one really knows. The bioethics industry may frown on that kind of experimentation – but I wonder how long abstract philosophical objections will last against the rising demand for organs, for vigorous flesh and blood, for extended life.

Of course there is another obstacle, and that is the nervous system. Surgeons do not now have the technology to cut off your head and sew it, functionally, on to a new body. They cannot reconnect big bundles of nerves. One or two nerves, here and there – yes, with microsurgical techniques. But a cable full of motor nerves connecting brain and bicep? No. An optic nerve connecting thousands of axons between eye and brain? No way. The spinal cord? Forget it.

One thing to bear in mind, however, is this: there are species on our planet, humble DNA-based life forms, that though very primitive compared to us nevertheless have the capability to regenerate very complex nerve systems very quickly. You can take, for example, a frog of the genus *Xenopus*, in its youth, and snip its optic nerve – a bundle of tens of thousands of wiry axons. Do that to a human, and you create permanent blindness in that eye. Do it to a young Xenopus and regeneration-mode genes turn on and the animal somehow, within a few weeks, re-establishes each and every one of those connections. The capability is there, left to us by nature.

When we are able to fix nerve bundles as well as lowly Xenopus can do, we will be able to do more than replace old organs in our bodies. We will be able to transplant limbs and eyes and make them fully functional. We will perhaps even be able to sever the spinal cord that connects our old brain to its old body and – slap – stick on a new body.

As for brain tissue, for nerve tissue – how do we regenerate that without destroying memories, hard-won instincts, the sense of self? How do we rejuvenate hardened, decayed networks of neurons without destroying the information held therein?

I don't know, of course. But I suspect that by the time we feel that we absolutely must answer such questions, we will be getting ready to move beyond transplants. We will be getting into the sensitive inner workings of cells, tinkering with DNA, turning disposable, mortal machines into ones that can run for ever.

PHASE THREE
FOREVER YOUNG

17

The Grey Gene

So now let us go to the genes.

And let us start with genes that commingle within families. Let us talk, as if we were on *Oprah*, about those confusing feelings cousins feel, growing up: boy cousins getting crushes on their girl cousins, girl cousins getting crushes on their boy cousins. Are these feelings . . . naughty? Are they sinful? Should a good Christian or Muslim or Darwinian disapprove?

The answer, you might say, is relative. Beyond the hard core of intrafamilial matings – brother-sister, father-daughter, mother-son – the morality becomes a bit fuzzy. That is to say, the taboo against first-cousin marriage is not something you find in every culture around the world. In many Third World cultures, in fact, such pairings are common and accepted, especially in rural areas where the local pool of prospective mates is small. Even in Western Europe and the USA first-cousin marriages were legal until five or six decades ago. Everybody did it. Albert Einstein married his first cousin. Even Charles Darwin married his first cousin – how's that for a sociobiological irony?

As Darwin might have suspected, a marriage like his ran the same kind of risk (albeit at one-fourth the level) that brother-sister marriages do.* It ran the risk of bringing together two copies of a mutant, bad form of a gene that had existed, as a single, harmless copy, in a common ancestor. It ran the risk of making a child who would suffer from disease for all her short life.

*   *   *

---

* The risk is doubled if the parent of one cousin is the identical twin of the parent of the other cousin.

Consider a woman who has a bad, non–functioning form of the gene known as CFTR. This bad gene is found on one of her two copies of chromosome 19. She inherited it from her father. On her other, slightly different copy of chromosome 19 (remember that humans have two copies of each chromosome, except for the X–Y chromosome pair men get) she has a good, functional form of the same gene, inherited from her mother. In other words, she is *heterozygous* for the bad CFTR gene. She has only one copy, out of a possible two. With the other, good form of CFTR doing its work in her cells she never notices anything wrong. But she passes the bad CFTR gene on to two sons. Both also inherit a good copy of the gene from their father, so they are heterozygous and healthy too. The sons each have a flock of children, of whom a few are again heterozygous for the bad gene. To all appearances, this is a healthy family tree.

Then disaster strikes. One daughter from one flock, who is heterozygous for the bad gene, elopes with her cousin, a son from the other flock, who as bad luck has it is also heterozygous. Of their four children two are heterozygous and healthy, and one has two good copies of the gene and thus is also healthy. But a fourth is *homozygous* for the bad gene, with two bad copies and no good copies, and thus completely lacks the function of CFTR in her cells.

This unfortunate girl gets the lethal disease that results from the lack of CFTR, the disease we call cystic fibrosis. She is in and out of hospitals with pneumonia all her short life, and dies at twenty–seven when the weakened wall of her pulmonary artery ruptures, and she drowns in her own blood.

Second–cousin marriage is less risky in this respect than first–cousin marriage – about four times less risky – but it's riskier than I'd like to try, even though it's legal. On the other hand, you can't really avoid risk, whenever you brings streams of genes together. Bad genes float around everywhere in the population. And if you go down deep enough into the genealogical records, for, say, English or Germans or Anglo–Saxonish Americans, or Japanese, you'll find that almost everyone is a 'cousin' – whether first cousin, fourth cousin, or fifteenth.

In the quiet town of Okayama, Japan, not far from Hiroshima, one wouldn't have had to dig very deep at all to connect two townspeople to a common ancestor. Especially not in the first decade of this century, when Shunichi Ishiguro met his future wife Michiko. They were not first cousins but they were probably closely related, for each had inherited a single copy of the same rare mutant gene from a common ancestor, probably a recent one.

They did not know of the existence of this mutant gene inside their cells when they married. They moved to the west coast of the United States, had nine children, and lived happily ever after – that is, dying in old age.

Six of the Ishiguro children were apparently normal and healthy. But three were quite strange. I am looking at a photograph of one now. Her name is Helen and she is standing almost naked on crutches, her face wearing a half-puzzled half-sad expression as a photographer takes her picture with a flash camera. She has almost undeveloped breasts, and thin arms and legs, and bandaged ankles, and she is only four feet eight. She weighs sixty-six pounds. Her hair is grey. She appears to be a small, elderly Japanese woman.

One day in 1960, four years before that picture was taken, Helen was referred by her family doctor to the University of Washington Hospital, near her home in Seattle. When she arrived she was suffering from severe ulcers on her feet and ankles and didn't know what to do about them. The doctor who examined her wasn't sure what to do about them either. The skin around her feet and ankles had a taut shine, almost a translucence, in which there was hardly any blood circulation. The skin was dying. The bones beneath were osteoporotic. Her whole body seemed to be greying and dying. But Helen explained, with her squeaky, hoarse, old-woman's voice, that she was only forty-four.

Helen, it turned out, had stopped growing when she was thirteen. At twenty-two she had noticed a haziness in her vision and was found to have a cataract in each eye; the cataracts were removed. Around this time her hair began to turn grey. By thirty-one she was clearly diabetic. She did not have juvenile diabetes; she had the kind that often struck people in their later years. Soon she began to undergo the hot flushes of menopause. This was not long after she had married. It didn't really matter; her libido had always been poor. She did not even have any pubic hair.

Helen's case attracted the attention of a group of researchers at the university. They asked Helen if she had any siblings who, like herself, had had such things as cataracts and grey hair at an early age. Yes, she said. She had two sisters who had been that way. One, Carol Ishiguro, had died at the age of thirty-one, apparently of diabetes. Carol had been even shorter than Helen and had weighed all of fifty pounds. She had had cataracted lenses removed from her eyes at age nine. She had stopped growing in her early teens. At the age of twenty-nine, when last examined by a doctor, she had already lost most of the hair on her head and also lacked both pubic hair and underarm hair. The doctor who then examined her diagnosed her with diabetes and a hormonally-caused dwarfism.

The other sister, Marion, was still alive, and the doctors coaxed her to come in for an examination. She weighed sixty-two pounds. The skin on her lower legs and feet was thin and dry and shiny. Her hair had turned grey when she was twenty and she had soon developed the rasping high-pitched voice that her sister Helen also had. At twenty-five she had lost the lenses of her eyes to cataracts. By her thirties her knee and ankle joints had begun to deteriorate and fuse, and she had open ulcers on her ankles and feet.

The group of researchers who studied the three Ishiguro sisters recognized that the women suffered from a rare genetic disease first described in the medical literature in 1904. It was called Werner's Syndrome and, like cystic fibrosis, it was a recessive disease. To get it, both a person's inherited copies of the responsible gene – one from the mother and one from the father – had to be dysfunctional. If your parents were not close relatives the chances that (a) each had one dysfunctional copy of the gene and (b) you inherited both those dysfunctional copies was roughly one in a million. If your parents were close relatives the chances were considerably higher, perhaps one in 5,000 to 10,000. Those odds were still very low. The mutant gene was terrible, but rare.

The group of researchers at the University of Washington – Charles Epstein, George Martin, Amelia Schultz and Arno Motulsky – described the three cases and summarized others in a forty-four-page review of the disease in the journal *Medicine* in 1966. They did not believe that Werner's was simply an abnormally speeded-up version of normal human ageing. But it was obvious to them that there were useful similarities. Most Werner's patients died before they reached fifty. Well before then they would suffer from cataracts, grey hair, osteoporosis, diabetes, a raspy voice, curvature of the spine, severe atherosclerosis and heart disease, and certain cancers.

As in the case of familial Alzheimer's at this time, scientists could do relatively little to find the Werner's gene, the gene whose functional absence in a person caused this rapid greying syndrome. The tools were simply not available. But young George Martin, the pathologist on the team of university researchers, collected blood samples from Helen Ishiguro during her hospital visits and skin samples from her body when she later died, in 1972. After establishing a culture from the cells he placed them in a bottle with a cryopreservative chemical, a 10 per cent solution of dimethyl sulphoxide. Then he placed the bottle of preserved cells in a canister of liquid nitrogen, as frigid vapour hissed at him from the top. Martin closed the canister and Helen Ishiguro's cells began their long hibernation.

Twenty-two years later, the same George Martin, now nearing seventy, now quite grey, opened the canister again. He took Helen Ishiguro's cells out of their liquid hibernation. He warmed them up, and fed them, and formed a new culture from the cells that had survived the long freeze. The year was 1994. The tools to manipulate those cells, to probe deep within their ribonucleic secrets, were now available. And a race was on to find the bad gene they contained.

18

The Race

Werner's Syndrome, like most pieces of knowledge, did not suddenly pop whole into the consciousness of medical science. When Otto Werner, a young eye doctor at a clinic in Kiel, Germany, wrote his ophthalmology thesis in 1904 on four siblings with early cataracts and grey hair and strange skin problems around the feet, gerontologists did not rise up and say, 'Aha! Werner's Syndrome!' There were no gerontologists back then. And medicine in 1904 had nothing like the cosmopolitanism and information–exchange that it has today.

It was not until 1934 that a couple of American scientists, B.S. Oppenheimer and V.H. Kugel, surveyed the scattered reports of cases like the ones Werner had described, and proclaimed the existence of 'Werner's Syndrome: a heredofamilial disorder with sclerodema, bilateral juvenile cataract, precocious graying of the hair and endocrine stigmatization'. Heredofamilial was a fancy way of saying that Werner's was inherited, genetic.

A few other major surveys occurred over the years, most notably one by S.J. Thannhauser at Tufts Medical School in 1945, and then the long paper by Charles Epstein and George Martin and their colleagues in 1966. But while there was general agreement on the features of Werner's, its clinical course and its sad outcome, the trail of knowledge ran into a wall when it approached the detailed genetics of the disease. Scientists simply did not know how to take lumps of tissue from Werner's patients, or syringes full of blood, and get down into the DNA of the cells and find the mutation responsible for the patients' apparently rapid ageing. The technology for doing that had not yet been invented.

Even so, there were a few early clues to what was going on, genetically, in Werner's Syndrome. For one thing the disease manifested all over the body, not just in one or two localized organs or tissues. The agony of Werner's was literally head to foot, from early grey hair down to cataracts, to underformed sex organs, to tearfully painful ulcers on the skin around the ankles, to corn-like hyperkeratotic growths near the toes. The gene that was not working in Werner's was a gene whose protein product ordinarily did something everywhere in the body.

—Or just about everywhere. It seemed that the only major ageing-related conditions Werner's did not accelerate were neurodegenerative diseases such as Alzheimer's and Parkinson's. Those were diseases in which neurons prematurely died. And neurons, in adults, were non-dividing cells. Which implied that Werner's primarily affected dividing cells: it fouled them up, somehow, during that critical, vulnerable phase when they shivered and split in two – when their seemingly endless chains of DNA, forty-six chromosomes of tightly, neatly coiled nucleic acids, uncoiled themselves and unwound themselves and surrendered themselves, naked, to a soup of enzymes and nucleotides from which a new copy of each chromosome would be synthesized, eventually resulting in the bubbling off of two cells where once had been one.

Werner's, one might have speculated, was a disease affecting the fidelity of the copying process. The cells of Werner's victims didn't divide properly; something happened to them, when they split in two, that was at least related to what happened during normal ageing.

In his early studies of Werner's patients, in the 1960s, George Martin like other scientists was aware of a newly described phenomenon known as the Hayflick Limit. Named for Leonard Hayflick, a cell biologist who had discovered this phenomenon in 1961, the limit referred to the fact that human cells, even when given seemingly ideal conditions in a lab culture dish, do not divide and make copies of themselves forever. After a certain number of divisions they simply stop dividing and become 'senescent' – gradually less efficient, eventually ceasing to function altogether.

The number of divisions before the limit is reached is different for different cell types in the body. But roughly speaking it is as if a clock has been started, somewhere at the time of the embryonic origins of every cell in every body. For a skin fibroblast cell from a newborn baby, say, the clock will have just begun ticking. It will still read early morning. In a culture dish, that newborn's cell will go through many more doublings than a similar cell taken from yourself, an adult – in whom that clock may be getting towards noon, or perhaps afternoon, or perhaps ten or eleven at night, depending on your age.

In 1969 George Martin found that cells from Werner's Syndrome patients reached their doubling limits, their Hayflick Limits, long before they should have. Their clocks, in effect, ran fast – way too fast.

And still no one knew why. Astronauts were up there, bouncing around on the moon, hopping grey dunes with their moon buggies, getting out their golf clubs and slicing 800-yard drives, and then stowing everything away and whooshing home to earth. And no one knew how to get into human DNA and find genes that had gone bad.

The tool that would allow scientists to begin doing that was invented in the early seventies but did not come into widespread use until a decade later. This tool, a very small tool, was the restriction enzyme. Restriction enzymes (in time scientists would discover hundreds of them) were enzymes found in certain bacteria. Their job was to cut up DNA from other, rival species of bacteria. Bacteria were always fighting it out with each other for food and space, and restriction enzymes – little cleavers 'restricted' to use against opponents' DNA – were one of their main weapons.

These enzymes cut only at certain nucleotide sequences, usually five or six bases long. For instance, an enzyme from the bacterium E. coli., known as EcoR1, always cut the sequence GAATTC just after the G, leaving loose ends that ended with G and AATTC. By adding a solution of this enzyme to a long stretch of DNA, say from an entire chromosome, one would cut the DNA into many smaller pieces, always at points where the sequence had been GAATTC. Some restriction enzymes cut sequences that were relatively common in human DNA, so that adding these enzymes to a sample of human DNA would result in very many pieces. Others only cut sequences that were rare; DNA cut with these enzymes would end up in a few large fragments. Scientists recognized that by applying different restriction enzymes to human DNA they could go through the entire genome, cutting it up into pieces, and then cutting select pieces into smaller pieces, and so on.

But here was the interesting thing. When DNA was cut up this way, the lengths of the resulting fragments differed from person to person, for the simple reason that the precise sequence of the genome differed from person to person. Sometimes in a gene a G (guanine) or an A (adenosine) would be missing, or a C (cytosine) would lie where a T (thymidine) should lie. Something like that. And this would mean that a given restriction enzyme might not cut where it did for another person's DNA. So the resulting gel blot of enzyme-snipped DNA fragments, lined up according to molecular weights, would be different for those two people.

With this tool in hand you didn't have to know the exact sequence of two people's genes to know that they were genetically different. All you had to do was look at the comparative lengths of their 'restriction fragments'. In areas of the genome where two people were very closely related – perhaps because they were first cousins – the fragments would tend to have the same lengths. In areas where they were less closely related, the fragments would tend to have different lengths. You could plot the statistical 'sameness' of their restriction fragment lengths on a chart. Where the chart had its little peaks was, roughly, where you could expect to find their genes to be the same. As one example, by comparing the members of a family who had a given genetic disease with those family members who didn't have the disease – and then doing the same for other families – one could eventually zero in on the area of the human genome where the diseased people in these families were always different from the healthy people.

Restriction fragment length analysis got you only so close to the location of a gene. To locate a gene precisely, one needed to be able to sequence all the As and Ts and Gs and Cs in a given stretch of DNA. In the early 1980s rapid and even automated DNA sequencing technologies became available, and scientists began to race each other to locate and sequence the genes for major hereditary diseases.

Muscular dystrophy was one of the first big targets, and a relatively easy one. It occurred only in males, but it could be inherited from females, which meant that it had to lie on the X chromosome. Women had two Xs, but men were out on a limb with one: if anything went wrong in their single X, they didn't have another copy for back-up.

Louis Kunkel, a biologist at Massachusetts General hospital who specialized in the study of the X and Y chromosomes, found a boy named Bruce Bryer, from Spokane, Washington, whose rare misfortune was to lack a large chunk of DNA from his X chromosome.

So large was this missing chunk that poor Bryer suffered from three separate genetic disorders: retinitis pigmentosa, chronic granulomatous disease, and muscular dystrophy. Which meant that his eyes didn't work, his immune system didn't work, and his muscles didn't work. As it had been with Helen Ishiguro and her sisters, Bryer's existence was a kind of sacrificial gift to science.

Louis Kunkel, to narrow the search for the muscular dystrophy gene, simply took Bryer's X chromosome, and used restriction fragment analysis – comparing Bryer's DNA to samples of normal DNA – to find where the chunk was missing. Now he knew the general area where the muscular dystrophy gene* lay, and could focus on that area, comparing the fragment lengths – and ultimately the actual nucleotide sequences – of more 'ordinary' muscular dystrophy sufferers to those from healthy individuals. Kunkel also knew, thanks to Bryer's missing chunk, where the genes for those other two genetic diseases lay. Within a couple of years of first sampling Bruce Bryer's DNA, Kunkel had identified the genes for both muscular dystrophy and chronic granulomatous disease. (Another team beat him to the retinitis pigmentosa gene.)

In 1986, in the midst of this early frenzy of gene-hunting, George Martin began an effort to increase his small collection of frozen blood and tissue cells from Werner's families. He added a freezer or two to his lab, and declared that his collection would henceforth be known as the International Registry of Werner's Syndrome. Martin intended to fill his freezers to the brim with blood and tissue samples from Werner's families. There was no point setting out on a search for a disease gene with an insufficient number of DNA samples to analyse. If you did that, you would likely end up running in circles, never able to zero in on the gene, because you lacked the statistical power to do so.

By the early 1990s Martin had collected enough samples to begin working with a team of genetics specialists led by Gerard Schellenberg, a University of Washington scientist who was about to head up a large gerontology lab at the Seattle Veterans Administration Medical

---

* Scientists, by the way, often confuse us by naming a gene not for the positive biochemical function it normally performs but instead for the disease that occurs when the gene is dysfunctional.

Center. Schellenberg had published some major papers on genes for early-onset Alzheimer's and apo-E4. Still in his late thirties, he was regarded as one of the world's best gene screeners.

But already it was clear that Martin and Schellenberg were the underdogs here. A rival team had formed, led by Dennis Drayna at the South San Francisco biotech giant Genentech Corp.

Drayna's big advantage was that he had access to the massive collection of Werner's samples kept by a University of Tokyo pathologist named Makoto Goto. Professor Goto, from his pathology lab down in the basement of Tokyo Metropolitan Otsuka Hospital, claimed to have seen 800 cases of Werner's, more than all other cases in the literature combined. Yet he had published relatively little about all these cases. His freezers were untapped mines of genetic gold.

By the time Martin and Schellenberg wrote to Goto, asking if he'd be willing to collaborate with them, it was too late. Genentech, some of whose scientists thought the gene for Werner's might hold the key to a future drug to slow ageing, already had struck a deal with him. So Drayna now had the formidable technical resources of Genentech plus an ample supply of Werner's family samples.

Gerard Schellenberg could only do the best he could with the precious samples he had, while George Martin went out and beat the bushes for more samples. The stakes were high. The Werner's gene, people now were starting to say, was the Holy Grail of ageing research.

Martin might have started his search for Werner's cases close to home. North America was quite a large place, population-wise. In 1990 a third of a billion people lived there. Surely in that vast expanse of humanity there would be pockets, little genetic islands, perhaps Eskimo villages in the Northwest Territories or banjo-twanging hollows in Appalachia, where centuries of inbreeding had produced some Werner's cases. Martin wanted Werner's cases from these inbreeding situations – 'consanguineous matings', in the genetic vernacular – because in such families one would be likely to find only a single kind of mutation to the Werner's gene, that mutation having come from a single ancestor linked to both sides of the family. If you had a case of Werner's arising from pure chance, in which a carrier with one mutant version of the gene had married a carrier with another mutant version of the gene, the confusion of mutations would make the analysis, which was already difficult, much more so.

The problem was, Martin could find almost no cases of Werner's in America. Where were the grey-haired twenty-year-old eskimos with ulcers on their ankles? Where were the teenage banjo savants with cataracts? Forget inbreeding; even random genetic shuffling, in which parents were carriers of the bad gene but were unrelated, should have generated a few hundred cases. Martin could find only a handful, and in most of those cases the patient had been born somewhere else, in rural Japan or in the Third World.

Now began George Martin's travels around the world in search of the grey gene. Let us imagine him as a low-key biomedical version of Indiana Jones, with a little medical bag in place of a bullwhip. And greying hair: for Doctor Martin himself was getting on now. The mystery of Werner's Syndrome had teased him throughout his career. Now these entwined entities – the Werner's mystery, Martin's career – were nearing their ends.

Martin went to India. To sweltering Lahore and Calcutta and New Delhi. To rural areas in the southern provinces, where not just cousin-to-cousin marriages but uncle-to-niece marriages were common, were usual, were quite OK. India had a huge population, and relatively well-trained doctors, especially ophthalmologists, whom Martin asked about early cases of cataracts with no apparent cause. Martin came back to the States with the cells from three affected families in his culture flasks. And soon he was off again, to France – fourteen pedigrees – to Mexico, and to Syria where he took blood and tissue samples from a huge, Werner's-afflicted clan in hot, dusty Damascus, as tinny loudspeakers wailed the call to prayer five times daily.

Meanwhile Martin's colleagues back in Seattle were beginning their search for the Werner's gene: taking Martin's samples of cells, and thawing them out, and transforming and multiplying the ones that had survived the long freeze. And adding detergents and protein-chewing enzymes to digest away everything but the DNA, leaving, after each such iteration, a speck of vital gene-stuff, a translucent dot of magic goo. And separating this goo with enzymes, and sorting the fragments by molecular weight, and sticking all the resulting data into a computer, and running software to analyse the fragment lengths and how they differed, person to person, and where the areas of greatest sameness lay in the samples from Werner's cases.

But before Martin and his group had really even started, the Goto/Genentech team struck.

Goto had taken cells from sixty-three people – thirty-one of them Werner's patients – in twenty-one families all over Japan. He had sent those cells across the Pacific to Dennis Drayna's lab at Genentech, where the cells were recultured and digested, leaving little globs of DNA for analysis.

In the summer of 1991 Drayna's group found three DNA fragments, all apparently on the short arm of chromosome 8, that tended to have the same length in the samples from the thirty-one people with Werner's. Drayna's lab sent a paper on this to *Nature*, which published it in February 1992.

The race was on, and the Goto/Drayna team was at least a step ahead of everybody else.

19

The Markers

Gerard Schellenberg, it should be said, was not the kind of man who became visibly stressed out in a competition like this. He looked, as one might have expected of a Schellenberg, quite Germanic, rustic Germanic in fact, like some dark-browed, bearded character from a Brothers Grimm tale, perhaps a blacksmith working a forge deep in some murky subalpine forest. But his voice was very American, very precise and intelligent, and very laid back. The voice of somebody who'd been there, done that, and didn't get ruffled.

Schellenberg had grown up near LA and had gone to university at UC-Riverside, getting his bachelor's degree in biochemistry in 1973. UC-Riverside, 1973: the peak of all that late-sixties early-seventies stuff. Let's be frank here: Schellenberg was the kind of guy – if you were going to take LSD for the first time, heavy duty, you'd want somebody like him around.

At the Seattle VA centre Schellenberg would stroll into the office six or seven every morning, wearing some kind of earth-shoe sandals, with socks, and baggy jeans, and maybe a loose sweater or a button-down shirt. The VA centre was perched on a hill and Schellenberg's office, up on the eighth floor, had a soothing view looking north-east over Seattle: the space needle, the glassy office district, the big gantries in the railyards by the wharf, and beyond that Elliot Bay, and the Olympic peninsula. Hard to get stressed out with a view like that massaging your eyes every day.

And yet – there was one subject whose mention could cause at least a hint of impatience to ripple across Schellenberg's features. That subject was Makoto Goto. The mysterious Goto, sitting on top of all those Japanese Werner's cases.

One day while I was in Schellenberg's office, having just met him, he said to me, 'There's a guy in Japan. Goto. He doesn't publish a lot.' Schellenberg now chuckled, very slightly, with what I imagined was a Schellenbergesque expression of exasperation. 'But he says he has records on eight hundred cases. And claims that five to ten per cent of them show dementia.' An important claim, that one, because if you look at all the others surveys of Werner's, you'll see that the common wisdom has long been that dementia is not one of the ageing-related diseases to which Werner's victims are prone. Heart disease, diabetes, cancer: yes. But dementia: no. For Goto to claim otherwise, without doing formal studies and publishing the results, is something that might reasonably cause consternation in fellow Werner's researchers. 'Now you know,' Schellenberg concluded with a smile, 'everything I know about what Goto's published on dementia in Werner's.'

When Schellenberg saw Goto and Drayna's *Nature* paper in February 1992, he quickly got his team to confirm the chromosome 8 result using their own techniques. They sent out a summary of their findings that April, in the form of a letter to the *Lancet*. At the end of the letter Schellenberg and his colleagues noted that 'refinement of the location of WSN [the Werner's Syndrome gene] will require additional families to be identified. For that purpose we have established an International Registry of Werner's Syndrome. This registry includes 61 subjects of eight countries . . .' George Martin's fax number was provided.

The message was clear enough, to anyone familiar with the race: The Schellenberg/Martin team were behind, and didn't have enough Werner's samples. They needed samples. They were crying out to the medical community: Send us samples!

Gene screening technology by now had moved beyond the use of simple restriction enzymes that cut fragments of varying lengths from a person's genome. Since around 1990 the modern gene-hunter instead had been checking 'repeat markers': short DNA sequences in which a given set of nucleotides is repeated a certain number of times.

For example, the sequence TTTA (thymidine, thymidine, thymidine, adenosine) occurs in a repeat form (TTTATTTATTTATTTA-TTTATTTA . . .) every so often in a given stretch of human genes, and in many cases the number of repeats at a given TTTA marker location (TTTATTTA = 2 repeats, TTTATTTATTTA = 3 repeats, and so on) varies slightly from person to person. One inherits it the same way one inherits other genetic information. And because one inherits a given form of a given repeat marker, gene screeners decided that they could use such markers as genetic signposts, more or less as they had used DNA fragments cut by restriction enzymes. They looked for areas of the genome where, for example, people with a genetic disease had the same lengths of repeat markers and people who didn't have the disease had different lengths.*

Genentech's Dennis Drayna, in his initial search for the Werner's gene in 1991, had looked at several kinds of repeat marker in the genomes of Japanese Werner's patients and their relatives. He looked at TTTA-repeat markers, TCTA-repeat markers, TTA-repeat markers, and at the most widely used of all repeat markers, the CA-repeat markers (CACACACA . . .). In all he checked markers at 156 separate locations spread across the human genome.

The skin and blood samples Drayna had received from Makoto Goto in Japan were mostly from rural inbred families in which first- or second-cousin marriages were common. Drayna knew that in such families Werner's would occur when an ancestral copy of the mutated Werner's gene found its way into both versions of whatever chromosome contained the gene.

Think of a chromosome as a single volume of a lengthy instruction manual. To reduce the effects of errors that might exist in a given manual, we are born with two copies of each manual. We have two copies of manual 1, two copies of manual 2, two copies of manual 3, and so on up to manual 23.†

Of course, these copies are not identical. At the time we originate,

---

* The technique used to pull out these repeat sequences was the polymerase chain reaction technique, or PCR. A 'primer' of nucleotides found next to the sought-for repeat sequence was added to the target DNA, and with a special enzyme and some heating and cooling cycles, pieces of the sought-for sequence were amplified out of the DNA until thousands or millions of them floated around in the solution, and they could easily be sorted by weight on a gel.

† Men, of course, have two different copies of 'chromosome 23' – we call them X and Y. But for genetic diseases it is relatively easy to tell when a mutation exists on chromosome X or Y because the resulting disease will have a higher prevalence in men. Most genetic diseases occur more or less equally in men and women because they are the result of mutations on the autosomes – chromosomes one to twenty-two – which exist in duplicate in all normal humans.

in our mothers' wombs, from sperm and egg, a tremendous, mysterious editorial rearrangement occurs so that for each copy of each manual, some pages are inherited from our father, and some from our mother; the result is that on any given page, the text in one copy comes from one parent, and the text in the other copy comes from the other parent. If our mother and father are closely related, we will find as we read through our separate copies of, say, manual 1, that there are long stretches of text that are exactly the same for both copies, that text having originated from our parents' common ancestor.

You could say, then, that Dennis Drayna's task, in searching for the one bad gene linking all these inbred Japanese Werner's victims, was to check manuals 1 to 22 for areas of text that were the same in both copies. In genespeak, he was looking for regions where the genetic information was homozygous. By noting these areas in Werner's victims and their near relatives, doing this for one affected family and then another and another, building up a database of perhaps dozens of families, Drayna and his computer could figure out which section of text (stretch of genes) in which manual (chromosome) was always homozygous – or much more homozygous than one would expect – in Werner's victims. Drayna knew that that piece of the genome would almost certainly be the one within which the Werner's gene lay: because the mutated Werner's gene had to exist homozygously, in both copies of its chromosome, for it to cause the disease.

Drayna, as he started his search, did not have the resources to sequence every genome of every individual in his sample, and then look for areas of homozygosity. That would be twenty-first century technology. Instead Drayna checked TTTA- and TCTA- and TTA- and CA- repeat markers at different places across the chromosomes, using the markers as little samples of text (asking: is a given marker in each copy of manual 1 the same? in manual 2? etc.), and recording the lengths of these markers for each of sixty-three people in twenty-one rural Japanese families.

Half of these people were Werner's victims and the rest were non-diseased relatives. As the data from Drayna's genetic analysing flowed through the Genentech computers, two markers quickly stood out. They were CA-repeat markers on chromosome 8. One was called D8S87, and the other ANK1 (because it lay within a gene that coded for a protein known as ankyrin). The statistics of Drayna's data showed that the lengths of these CA-repeat markers were the same for most of the Werner's victims. In genespeak, these markers had significantly increased homozygosity.

Eventually Drayna found that three other markers on chromosome 8 also showed increased homozygosity in Werner's victims. That meant that the Werner's gene lay somewhere in the midst of all these markers. Looking at the homozygosity values for the five markers, Drayna estimated that the Werner's gene lay nearest to D8S87 and ANK1, which were on chromosome 8's short arm, 'p', somewhere around band number 12. Efforts now could focus on that neighbourhood: 8p12.

Up in Seattle, Schellenberg's team was falling behind. But at least they now had access to some Japanese samples, thanks to a collaboration George Martin had established with an Osaka University gerontologist named Tetsuro Miki. The Schellenberg team badly needed those Japanese samples; Japan's population was by far the richest ore a Werner's scientist could mine. Japanese seemed to have an unusually high incidence of Werner's, and their fast-ageing society was also unusually gerontology-conscious: cases of Werner's were seldom overlooked.

Using Miki's samples, Schellenberg's team of gene screeners checked repeat markers on chromosomes 1 to 22, recording those for which their Werner's victims were homozygous, and comparing the frequencies with which certain variants appeared among Werner's victims and unaffected control individuals. As Drayna had done, they quickly zeroed in on the CA-repeat markers D8S87 and ANK1, around chromosome 8p12.

By then, Drayna's team had already taken the hunt for the Werner's gene a step further. They were working along two main tracks: First, checking known genes in the 8p12 region for any whose dysfunction might explain Werner's Syndrome; and second, looking for new repeat markers in the 8p12 region that could be used to narrow the location of the elusive Werner's gene.

The first track didn't really lead anywhere. The two genes Drayna's group checked didn't seem likely to be the gene whose mutation caused Werner's.

But on the second track, looking for new markers in the 8p12 region, the Genentech team had some success. Winston Thomas, a scientist in Drayna's lab, found a CA-repeat marker on chromosome 8 for whom most people in the Japanese population were heterozygous. Most Japanese, in other words, had two copies with different lengths. But for Japanese Werner's victims, the two copies of that marker almost always had the same lengths. Of the twenty-one Werner's samples studied in Drayna's lab, all but one were homozygous for the new marker. That meant that the new marker – they named it WT251, the WT for 'Winston Thomas' – was very close to the Werner's gene, probably on its very doorstep.

In the six months after Schellenberg and his colleagues read Winston Thomas's paper in *Genomics* their Seattle lab buzzed with activity as more samples came in, more markers were checked. They were finding that the disease wasn't as simple as they had hoped. The kinds of markers that were linked to the Werner's gene in the Japanese population didn't link as well to Caucasian Werner's cases. Which implied that the mutations in the Japanese Werner's patients had were different from those in Caucasian Werner's patients. Worse, Schellenberg's team concluded that the Caucasian patients themselves probably did not all have the same kind of mutation. In all, it seemed, there were at least several mutations out there that resulted in Werner's Syndrome. Several different ways that nature, cruel nature, had disabled the normal, healthy gene.

Early in 1994 Schellenberg's lab sent out three long papers, two to *Genomics* and one to the *American Journal of Human Genetics*. The papers described their work so far and concluded that the best marker for Werner's so far was WT251 – now known, more anonymously, as D8S339 – although that marker was probably not in the same place Winston Thomas had thought it was in. Instead of being on the side of the Werner's gene closer to the centre of chromosome 8, the *centromere*, as Thomas and Drayna had first announced, it now was thought more likely to be on the side closer to the end of that arm of chromosome 8 – closer to the chromosome's *telomere*.

In any case, the area of unknown DNA within which the Werner's gene lay was still too large to begin sequencing. It was at least eight megabases long: eight megabases being 8 million nucleotides, 8 million individual As and Gs and Ts and Cs. Only when someone had narrowed the gene to an area of about 1 million megabases could sequencing – the step by step decoding of nucleotides, to determine the text of the actual gene – actually begin.

As Schellenberg and his team contemplated this abyss that separated them from the end of the race, they also wondered, worriedly, what Drayna's lab was up to. Drayna and Genentech and Goto had put nothing into the literature since their *Genomics* paper in early 1993. Had they quit for some reason, or were they running silent to keep Schellenberg from catching up?

Eventually Schellenberg found out what had happened: Drayna had quit Genentech to join a startup biotech company, Mercator Genetics. His lab had turned to other things, and Genentech, for whatever reason, had abandoned the Werner's race.

That might have been good news for Schellenberg and his team. But there was other news, announced one day by a fax that spooled in from across the Pacific, in Japan. It was a news release announcing the formation of a new Japanese biotech company, Agene. The mission of this new company was to find and clone the Werner's gene and to use that information to make some kind of miracle anti-ageing drug. The Japanese were dead serious about this. They had several tens of millions of dollars in funding, including government funding, and they had twenty-plus people working in a new and well-furnished Tokyo laboratory. And they had Makoto Goto, and all his samples. And they were working hard. And they were not going to publish anything until they had won the race.

Meanwhile Schellenberg and his own hard-working postdocs and technicians and fellow scientists still stared out over that eight-megabase abyss. How the hell were they going to get across it? Even laid-back Schellenberg, looking back on this phase of the race, would remember: 'It was kinda scary.'

Chang-En Yu, one of the postdocs in Schellenberg's lab, was a young Taiwanese who had gone from Taipei to grad school at the University of Oklahoma. When I asked him how he'd liked dusty Oklahoma, compared to bustling Taipei, he remembered happily that it was quiet, peaceful.

It was not so quiet and peaceful in Schellenberg's lab. In addition to the gut-knotting stress of the race with the mysterious Goto, there was the matter of ambient noise.

Chang-En's office was a small space tucked into a corner of the lab, beneath galvanized aluminium air-ducts that throbbed almost painfully with the low-frequency pulses of their blowers. HOMMMMMMMMMMMMMMMMMMM. Chang-En had to keep earplugs in his ears – or headphones plugged into a Walkman tape player – just to stay sane in there. The view out the window was nice, though. Snowcapped Mount Rainier, seventy miles away. When it wasn't raining.

Chang-En Yu had been lead author on one of the papers published in that flurry of correspondence coming from Schellenberg's lab in early 1994. His paper had announced that Japanese Werner's cases were inordinately likely (a) to have a certain form of the D8S339 marker and also (b) to have certain forms of two CA-repeat markers within a nearby gene, known as GSR, which coded for an enzyme known as glutathione reductase. Chang-En's data suggested that the Werner's gene lay within 500,000 to a million kilobases of D8S339, though it wasn't clear which direction. The lab didn't have enough markers in the area to show a clear pattern of linkage becoming weaker as the distance from the gene area increased. All they had were markers a few million base pairs out which showed no linkage. The gap between those no-linkage markers, either side of the gene, was the eight-megabase abyss.

Chang-En Yu, working with two other Schellenberg postdocs – Junko Oshima and Ying-Hui Fu – focused on that eight-megabase region and tried to find more repeat markers that showed less variability in Werner's cases than in controls. It was a painstaking process: amplifying fragments of the eight megabases of DNA to find CA repeats, then checking the lengths of the repeats on agarose gels, then running the data through a computer to look for patterns, for differences between cases and controls.

Summer came – the dry season – then faded into rainy autumn. The number of useful markers within the eight-megabase region slowly grew. And as they did, Chang-En and the others began to see the signs of 'recombination events' within this region: places where a switch suddenly occurred between a chromosome segment inherited from the father, and one from the mother (or vice versa).

Two of these recombination events effectively marked the ends of a 1.3-megabase stretch within which the markers all showed strong linkage to Werner's cases. Outside this 1.3-megabase stretch the markers showed little or no linkage.

This was cause for celebration. The eight-megabase abyss had been

narrowed down to a fraction of its original size. 1.3 megabases was
manageable enough that the lab could now start sequencing DNA,
looking in detail at all the nucleotides.

'We knew then,' Schellenberg would later remember, 'that this
project was doable.'

But the word doable, in this context, merely meant that it was
humanly possible with present technology. It definitely wasn't going
to be easy.

To get some idea of the problem, imagine that your task is to find a
particular kind of misprint that you know exists – somewhere – in a few
dozen copies of a novel. It's a wordy, meandering novel, a Tom Clancy
novel, a great leaden slab of a book. Now imagine that the particular
kind of misprint you're looking for is so bad that it drastically changes
the ending to the story, in a way that the author didn't intend. The
bad guys win, or something like that.

Now imagine, in addition, that the novel is written in a language you
don't fully understand; you can understand individual characters, and
words, but not usually their meanings in combination. And in each of
those mutant copies of this giant Tom Clancy novel there are misprints
galore, not just the one that has ruined the ending. The only way you
know that the ending has been ruined, in those few dozen copies, is
that the people who read them tend to throw the book down in disgust
when they're only half-way through.

Well, one thing to do, in searching for this key misprint, would
be to simply take all the pages of the book, and run them through
a document scanner, soaking up all the As and Gs and Cs and Ts,
doing that for the books you know have the strange misprint as well
as for a selection of the ones that don't. And then have a computer
analyse the differences. Eventually it will be clear that all the mutant
books have one single misprint in common, one that isn't found in the
normal versions of the book. Simple, right?

Not really. There are too many random, minor misprints in all the
books, and too few of the mutant books with the wrong ending, for
such an easy analysis to work. And there is more than one misprint
that spoils the book by having the bad guys win. There is, in fact, a
whole group of these fatal misprints, presumably all occurring around
the same page.

To make matters even more difficult, these books are all written in invisible ink. So you can't use a simple scanner. You have to go through, page by page, applying expensive chemicals to each page to tease out the letters. And then you feed everything into your computer, and hope for the best – and also hope that the Japanese, who are doing the same thing but have more money, don't beat you.

Schellenberg's basic strategy was to methodically sequence the DNA within the 1.3-megabase Werner's-linked region, and to look for genes in the region, and to check these genes for variants that occurred in Werner's cases but didn't occur in controls.

The raw sequencing was done at a local biotech house, Darwin Molecular. Schellenberg's lab workers would isolate DNA segments from the 1.3 megabase stretch, snap them into easy-to-handle molecular modules that grew inside bacteria, and courier packed lab dishes of the stuff across town to Darwin, whose workers would put the clones through big sequencing machines, and then send back computer disks, a couple of weeks later, with the genetic sequence of the segment they'd been given.

With these disks in hand, Chang-En Yu and Ying-Hui Fu began to analyse the raw DNA sequences for evidence of genes.

As with everything else in this race, finding genes was harder than it sounded. One thing Chang-En and Ying-Hui tried was to check sequences against databases of known genes.* In this way they found several known genes in the 1.3 megabase region. But when they compared the lengths of these known genes in Werner's cases and controls, they found no consistent differences. The gene whose dysfunction caused Werner's was not a known gene.

So Chang-En and Ying-Hui tried another method: running the raw sequence data through a software programme called GRAIL, which was supposed to detect evidence of genes – sequences that would express themselves as amino acids, and not just lie inert within the genome – amid all the As and Ts and Gs and Cs. The problem with GRAIL was that it didn't work very well. Nine times

---

* Human DNA is not a neat chain-link of genes, one after another. Between genes and even within genes there lie stretches, sometimes very long stretches, of apparently inactive DNA known as introns. DNA that is part of a gene and expresses its information (in the from of RNA, and from RNA to amino-acids which make proteins) is known as an exon.

out of ten, the 'gene' it found was nothing more than genomic fluff, and the search for differences in that gene, between Werner's cases and controls, led nowhere. Sometimes Schellenberg and the others wondered whether GRAIL wasted more time than it saved.

So Chang-En and Ying-Hui used yet another method, in parallel with the first two. They checked the raw DNA sequence data against a database – the 'expressed sequence tag' (EST) database – of many of the expressed sequences (that is, not the inert sequences) in the human genome.

And the days went by, and the work went on.

And one day, late in 1995, Schellenberg heard the news he had long dreaded.

The Japanese had found the Werner's gene. The mysterious Goto, with his biotech partners, had triumphed. Someone in the Goto camp had told somebody else, and that person had told somebody else, and now the news was spreading everywhere, over the Internet.

Schellenberg, and Chang-En Yu, and Ying-Hui Fu, and every-body else, kept working. Watching the Internet, watching their fax machine, waiting for confirmation of the bad news. They knew it was possible that the Japanese findings were a false alarm. That often happened in searches for genes. No matter how promising a piece of data might appear, it always had to be confirmed again and again before one could really believe in it.

Meanwhile the days were getting shorter, and rainier, and darker.

One dreary afternoon, just around the winter solstice of 1995, a couple of days before Christmas, Chang-En Yu came out of the darkroom behind his little office with the humming overhead ducts. He was looking at a photograph of an agarose gel he had run that morning.

The fragments arranged in lanes on the gel were pieces of DNA from some of the Werner's cases and controls. The DNA fragments were fragments of a gene, or piece of a gene, that he had found on the expressed-sequence tag database. Chang-En, as on most days, was merely carrying out the rote work of checking these fragments for differences between Werner's cases and controls. In this case, the gel contained fragments pulled from the DNA of three Japanese Werner's families, one Caucasian Werner's family, and several controls.

On the gel, the fragments had been incubated with phosphorescent molecules, and their tiny glows showed up on polaroid film as white rectangles on a field of blackness. If the fragments were all the same length, then they would have been arranged in a neat side-by-side row across the bottom of the gel, at a position that indicated the length of these fragments: about 1,000 base-pairs. But the little white rectangles were not arranged in a neat side-by-side row. The rectangles belonging to two of the Japanese families were both below the others, indicating that the gene fragments, in these cases, were missing about ninety-five base pairs – about 10 per cent of their normal length. In other words, the Werner's cases in those two separate families each had the same mutation in some gene at the heart of the Werner's-linked region.

Chang-En was still holding the photograph of the gel, there under the humming air ducts in his office, when Schellenberg happened to walk in. In his thick Chinese accent Chang-En nervously said to Schellenberg: 'I think we might have something interesting here.'

20

The Gene Cleaner

Victory was not sudden; it was gradual, a process of checking results, extending them, overcoming residual doubts like an army rooting out stragglers from enemy bunkers and trenches. When Schellenberg and his team heard that the Japanese result had after all been spurious, a false alarm, they still were not certain that the long struggle was over. Only after another month of adrenal, blurred, twelve-hour days did they establish to their own satisfaction that the DNA fragment missing in the two Japanese Werner's cases was a single, 95 base-pair exon from a 5,200 base-pair gene. The other Werner's cases all had other deletions or small but significant mutations in that same gene.

It was the Werner's gene, and despite the thorny mystery in which it had once been wrapped it had how been found, conclusively, by methodical scientists wielding new and powerful technology. When I later asked Schellenberg what it had been like to find the gene – like winning the lottery? – he chuckled: 'Yeah, like winning the lottery. Except we bought all the tickets.'

Schellenberg's group found four separate mutations in the gene, each running in one or more Werner's families. The normal version of the gene, when its sequence was compared to those of other genes from humans and other animals, obviously belonged to a family of genes for helicases: housekeeping enzymes that live in the nuclei of cells.

It was a result that made sense. Human DNA is very long, and to squeeze forty-six chromosomes worth of this DNA – a couple of feet, if you could unwind it all – into the nucleus of a cell is not a simple matter. The DNA is not just wound into a double helix, like a twisted ladder. It is wound into a double helix and then wound again, folded over and twisted, and wound some more.

Take a coiled phone handset cord and start twisting it and you'll get the idea.

Now, all this twisting and winding has to be undone periodically, for example whenever a cell decides to divide and make two cells. Although this is a routine event it is also a moment of cellular chaos and crisis. Billions of chemical bonds are broken apart and must be put back together again. Large and small errors can occur, and these errors can lead to cancer, to cell death, or to a slow cellular degeneration as key proteins fail to do their work. Helicases, as far as cell biologists can tell, are there to reduce these errors. They are there to keep your DNA clean when it unwinds itself apart and later winds itself back together.

Obviously, then, a malfunction in a key helicase could have an enormous impact on the long-term integrity of your DNA. Lacking that helicase, errors would accumulate more quickly in your genes. As Schellenberg would write, sitting in front of his computer in his office high over Seattle, composing the paper that would appear in *Science* two months later: 'The consequence of the Werner's Syndrome defect in DNA metabolism may be the accumulation of DNA mutations, leading to the age-related diseases observed in Werner's Syndrome ... Whatever the specific mechanisms involved in the Werner's Syndrome [disease], identification of the Werner's Syndrome gene now provides evidence that at least some components of 'normal' aging and disease susceptibility in late life may be related to aberrations in DNA metabolism.'

In other words, if you could keep your genes clean, you might live longer, perhaps a lot longer.

There are many other reasons, besides defects in helicases, that DNA accumulates mutations throughout life.

One of these other reasons is the free radical, especially the oxygen free radical. A free radical is a molecule – hydrogen peroxide, for example – with an unpaired electron in an outer orbit. The unpairedness of that electron makes the molecule chemically unstable; it fiercely wants to bind to things and react with them. Oxygen free radicals bind to, and damage, just about everything in the body, from fatty proteins and carbohydrates to DNA.

Mitochondria, the little bacteria-like power plants that live inside cells, are one of the greatest producers of oxygen free radicals. As part of their energy production process, mitochondria burn oxygen. (This, by the way, is one big reason why we breathe: to supply oxygen to our mitochondria.) The oxygen arrives in the form O_2, and most of it is converted to the molecule H_2O – water. But as with any combustion engine, this burning of oxygen isn't 100 per cent efficient. Some of the oxygen ends up in free-radical form, damaging the DNA of mitochondria as well as the DNA further away inside the nucleus. The fairly direct relationship between energy-burned and free-radicals-produced may explain why laboratory rats that are forced to eat low-calorie diets – and thus burn less energy – live significantly longer, on average, than they would otherwise.

Free radicals also form as by-products of toxins (e.g. in cigarette smoke) as they are broken down inside the body. And they are probably the major reason why ultraviolet light speeds the ageing of skin and promotes cancer: UV energy is strong enough to knock electrons from their molecular orbits, thus creating unpaired-electron molecules – free radicals – which create unwanted mutant compounds, great organic carbuncles, on nearby DNA.

Mutations to DNA also can happen more or less spontaneously, every time a cell divides, simply because organic things don't work perfectly. In any case, evolution has generously provided us with strong repair and maintenance mechanisms – 'housekeeping' mechanisms – such as helicases that keep DNA from tearing and tangling when it unwinds; and translation enzymes that manage the conversion of DNA information to RNA information to proteins; and repair enzymes that can recognize a mutation and resynthesize the correct sequence.*

But again, these mechanisms never work perfectly. Errors accumulate, and perhaps eventually they affect the genes that code for these housekeeping functions themselves. Within a cell, a vicious circle begins, as mutations in housekeeping genes result in less efficient housekeeping, and a greater overall mutation rate, which causes more mutations to housekeeping genes, or

---

* DNA is double-stranded, with essentially the same information encoded on each strand. Thus a mutation to one strand can usually be fixed by making use of the correct information on the other, unmutated strand. Double-strand errors are, naturally, harder to fix.

other deleterious changes to the cell, and so on, and so on, as the cell decays and dies. If the cell is part of a non-dividing family of cells, such as neurons, this will be the end of the line; the dead cell won't be replaced. If the cell is part of a population of still-dividing cells, such as epithelial cells that line the gut, its siblings with more intact DNA will survive and take its place – but the process of decay will continue inexorably in all such cells until Hayflick Limits are reached and senescence sets in.

As I mentioned a few chapters ago, the cells of Werner's Syndrome victims reach their Hayflick Limits far sooner than the cells of the rest of us do. Something about Werner's DNA causes it to take, with every cellular doubling, a comparatively giant step toward senescence and death. But even if you don't have Werner's – even if you are spry and sharp and still have a mop of hair at eighty – the dark wall of senescence is out there waiting for you.

The immediate cause was discovered in the 1970s. The central junction of the arms of a chromosome (which is roughly X- or Y-shaped) is called the centromere, while the loose ends are called the telomeres. The telomeres contain monotonous repeat sequences of DNA: TTAGGG on one strand, and the complementary sequence AATCCC on the other. These repeat sequences seem inert. They just go on, repeating themselves hundreds of times. They seem like junk.

But they are not junk. Telomeres are precious to a cell. They are something like Teflon. Without them protecting the ends of chromosomes, those ends would all stick together when their DNA unwound, and that would keep the cell from dividing successfully.

At least in part because of this (our understanding of telomeres is in its infancy), telomeres serve as a kind of biological clock for most cells. Every time a cell doubles, its chromosomes lose bits of their telomeres. So the telomeres on the two daughter cells' chromosomes are a bit shorter than they were in the original mother cell. Some of those TTAGGG/AATCCC repeats have been ripped away in the hurly-burly of cellular division. Eventually, when a cell has divided many times and the telomere repeat sequences have been whittled entirely or almost entirely away, the cell stops dividing. It is now in the mode that cell biologists call senescence. It has reached its Hayflick Limit.*

Now, some cells in the body (sperm-producing cells, egg cells) are known as germline cells. They are god-like cells and, starting from their original form (a sperm-fertilized egg), they spin off all the ordinary mortal cells that live and die in the body, but they themselves – the germ cells – apparently never lose the capability to stop dividing, and they go on to the next generation. Think of an egg cell: when fertilized by a sperm cell within the body of a mother it becomes an embryo and starts to divide. Let's assume a daughter is being produced here. In one of its divisions the embryonic cell-group splits off another egg cell, which then produces thousands more, and these seed the ovaries of the daughter, and through the same process† those eggs go on to seed the ovaries of her daughter, and so on through history.

The telomeres of these egg cells never shorten to stumps, but instead maintain a length of about 15,000 bases. For many years scientists wondered why – what process in these cells kept the telomeres long? – but then in 1984 Elizabeth Blackburn and Carol Greider at UC-Berkeley discovered an enzyme they called telomerase. This magic enzyme, they observed, relengthens telomeric DNA after every shortening caused by chromosomal division.

When it became clear that this was what telomerase did, it suggested an obvious hypothesis: if you could somehow insert telomerase into

---

* At the time of writing, no one knows why Werner's cells lose their telomeres more quickly than other cells. One possible reason is that the faulty helicase, during cellular division, allows errors and breaks in the telomeres along with other DNA errors. It is also possible that this speeded-up damage to telomeres is the major cause of disease in Werner's cases.

† Though much remains to be learned about germline cells it is widely assumed that most accumulated DNA defects in them either result in cell death or are repaired during meiosis, the mixing of sperm and egg chromosomes at conception. In any case, something happens to restore telomeres, and, perhaps, to regain some DNA defects, when a germline cell mixes with its opposite number (a sperm cell, an egg cell) to form an embryo. A recent cloning experiment at the University of Massachusetts shed a weird light on this process. Researchers there took a fibroplast cell from a foetal calf, let it double to its Hayflick limit in a lab dish, and then fused it with a calf egg cell from which the DNA (the yolk, so to speak) had been removed. The 'aged' fibroplast DNA, now surrounded by the walls of an egg cell, apparently decided it was an embryo. Its telomeres were somehow restored and it started to form – and eventually did form – a new and so far healthy cloned calf.

mortal cells, perhaps it would render them god-like, immortal. In other words, telomerase might be some kind of enzymatic fountain of youth.

Motivated by this kind of thinking, a team at Geron Corp. in San Francisco, led by Calvin Harley, has been doing telomerase work since the late 1980s.

One thing that they and others eventually recognized was that the gene for telomerase already exists within mortal, Hayflick-Limited cells; it just lacks a key component and thus is normally dormant. Harley's goal has been to find a way to switch on the usually-dormant telomerase gene in ordinary mortal cells, to let the cells live longer, perhaps for ever.

In early 1998, Harley and his group, working with colleagues at the University of Texas Southwestern in Dallas, made a big media splash with a paper in *Science*. After inserting a small gene into normal, telomere-shortening cells to switch on the production of telomerase, they observed that the altered cells did indeed keep dividing beyond the normal limits. With their telomeres kept long and strong by telomerase, they reached at least 50 per cent more doublings by the time Harley's group wrote up their results.

As if propelled by that very number, Geron's stock price also shot up 50 per cent. And that was easy to understand. Harley and Co., in their paper, made clear that they considered this more than just an interesting lab result. 'Cellular senescence,' they wrote, 'is believed to contribute to multiple conditions in the elderly that could in principle be remedied by cell life-span extension in situ.' In other words, the right dose of some telomerase-based drug could make your cells young again.

But perhaps that is too good to be true. For one thing, relatively little is known about telomeres and telomerase and their ultimate reasons for existence. They do have reasons for existence, but presumably Evolution did not create them as a simple on/off switch for mortality.

Probably the most widely accepted hypothesis about the function of telomeric shortening is that it serves to limit the chances that bad mutations, especially cancerous mutations, will occur in cellular DNA. Remember that every cellular division is a moment of crisis for DNA. All those organic bonds must be broken and then put back together again. In fact, each time a cell divides to form two daughter copies some errors will occur in the resulting cells' DNA and will not be repaired successfully. That is statistically inevitable. And the more times a cell divides in its replicative lifetime, the greater the chance it will incur errors that push it into uncontrolled, cancerous mode.

If cells have no replicative limits, then the chances they will go cancerous are greater. Telomerase, applied to normal, mortal cells of advanced age and creaky DNA to force them to continue dividing, may simply be a recipe for cancer. In fact, the first place researchers found telomerase in human cells was in cancer cells. To stay or become cancerous, cells must either switch on telomerase production or re-lengthen their telomeres through some other mechanism. Unsurprisingly, then, much of the buzz about telomerase in the scientific community has been about finding ways to switch it *off*, in cancer cells.

Another thing to bear in mind is that several key cell types in the body are essentially non-dividing throughout one's life. They reach their limits early, yet they do not die young. I am talking about neurons, for example, and cells within the heart muscles. Even after these cells reach their Hayflick Limits and become 'senescent' they can continue functioning, well, for about a century. And except in extraordinarily rare cases they do not become cancerous. So the loss of telomeric DNA doesn't necessarily mean that a cell is going to die soon; but it does mean that the chances of cancer are drastically reduced.

At the same time, it should be borne in mind that the loss of telomeres, the Hayflick Limit, is not something that suddenly hits us all when we reach old age, throwing our cells down the slope of decay. George Martin once did a study of the doubling potential of cells, comparing those from infants to those from older people. He found that the skin fibroblasts of people in their eighties – that is, people on the actuarial brink of death – still had significant doubling potential left, in fact about 60 per cent of the doubling potential of the infant cells. Adding telomerase might have had no effect at all on such cells, which obviously had most of their telomeres intact and therefore were ageing for reasons other than the loss of telomeric DNA.

On the other hand, it could be that even intermediate telomere loss, as seen in these elderly fibroblasts, sets off some kind of programmed decay process. Cellular senescence isn't something that happens all at once; it is gradual, involving a number of slow changes in the cell. It might also be the case that senescence in a small fraction of a given population of cells has effects (for example, reduced repair potential) that are the same as what we know as ageing.

Moreover, regarding cancer, it is not clear that rebuilding telomeres with telomerase will inevitably lead to the growth of tumours. Germline cells, which use telomerase to maintain their ability to divide, do not seem inordinately prone to cancer. Still, that might be because germline cells have sturdier DNA-repair kits than mere mortal cells do. In any case the human cells dosed with telomerase in the Geron experiments did not suddenly turn tumourous. But they might, eventually, as Harley and company admitted in their paper: 'The long-term effects of exogenous telomerase expression on telomere maintenance and the life span of these cells remain to be determined in studies of longer duration.'

Which is to say: more experiments are needed. In the meantime it seems unlikely that telomerase, a specialized enzyme for a special class of cells, can serve as an instant lifespan-increaser on its own. Certainly I would not want to artificially extend the doubling life of my own cells with telomerase – not unless I had first corrected all the underlying DNA errors my cells had accumulated.

DNA is far from being the only thing that degrades with ageing. Take bones: they have some self-repair capability, more so when they are younger, but as they age they develop apparently irreversible chemical changes and wear out, and become brittle, and tinkering with DNA night work for younger bones, to keep them young, but it isn't going to be an easy way to make old people orthopedically youthful again. To do that we'll probably have to transplant new bone in, either lab-grown or synthetic. The same probably goes for our teeth*, and the tympanic membranes of our ears, and the lenses of our eyes: it will probably be easier, in older people, to transplant than to attempt some kind of regrowth or rejuvenation inside the body.

If much of ageing is caused by the build-up of errors in DNA within cells, much also is caused by errors in non-DNA material, outside the cell. Or perhaps errors isn't the right term. Better to call it a build-up of insoluble proteins and other unwanted formations – gunk – such as amyloid plaques, and cholesterol plaques, and the age-pigment (lipofuscin) that inevitably accumulates in non-dividing cells.

Probably the largest single part of the gunk problem is what is known as 'cross-linking': the more or less random binding of proteins

---

* Perhaps some cell biologist will figure out a drug that will let us grow unlimited sets of teeth beyond the two ('baby teeth', 'adult teeth') we normally are given.

to other proteins in a process that reduces elasticity and generally reduces function. The collagen fibres in skin, for example, become increasingly cross-linked with age. Pinch a fold of skin on the back of your hand and then let go and watch it settle back. Did it settle back slowly? If so, your collagen is already quite cross-linked; your skin is well aged.

Glycosolation is a term for what is probably the most significant form of cross-linking, which involves the attachment of ordinary proteins to sugar (glyco-) molecules. Glycosolated proteins begin to form a sticky mess that attracts other proteins and sugars. Effectively a slow-motion form of cooking, it's what turns a fresh red steak brown in the refrigerator.

It gradually turns your own meat brown, too, despite the best efforts of your body. As glycosolation reactions proceed they eventually form compounds called 'advanced glycosolation end-products' – AGEs, for short. AGEs are bits of gunk that slow and stiffen the ageing body, and can't be removed by the normal housekeeping mechanisms nature has given us. AGEs harden cartilage and the walls of arteries and the lenses of eyes; they help thicken and stiffen membranes and collagens in muscles, the retinas, the kidneys, the skin, and so on. The process is speeded up in diabetics, who suffer from frequent overloads of blood sugar, but it happens anyway, more slowly, in people who are not diabetic. If you have always suspected that eating sweets is bad for you, but lacked deep reasons, look no further: gorging on sweets may well hasten the ageing process through glycosolation.

Not that you can completely avoid glycosolation. Along with DNA errors, and the mechanical wearing of bones and teeth, and the damaging free radicals created as cells burn energy, glycosolation is an inevitable by-product of Life. You can't prevent it; you can only look for ways to slow it or reverse it after it has begun.

Fortunately it already seems possible to do this. A few years ago collaborating scientists at the small biotech house Alteon Inc., in Ramsey, New Jersey, and at the privately-endowed Picower Institute in Manhasset, New York, developed a compound they called pimagedine ('pih-MAH-djeh-deen'). Pimagedine interferes with the cross-linking process, slowing it down. In early clinical trials with diabetes patients, pimagedine seems among other things to have lowered the levels of harmful cholesterol (LDL) in their bloodstreams. That in turn lends a little support to one of the current theories about

LDL cholesterol and vascular disease: The theory is that LDL in older patients is increasingly modified with AGEs, which prevent the LDL from being cleaned up by the normal, healthy mechanisms of the body; instead the LDL molecules stay too long in the system, and gunk up the walls of arteries.* So pimagedine, if all goes well in its continuing clinical trials, could be good not just for diabetes but also for preventing heart disease and stroke in the ageing population generally.

Alteon and Picower also have been at work on AGE-breakers, compounds which are meant not to slow glycosolation but to reverse it, to break up all those chains of glucose and protein that have clotted your tissues over the years. The two groups of scientists announced their first AGE-breaker in *Nature* in the summer of 1996, reporting that it had the ability to dissolve glycosolation cross-links in the tissues of rats. Since that paper the collaborating biochemists, led by Jack Egan at Alteon and Peter Ulrich at Picower, have devised an even better compound, to which they've given the temporary name ALT-711, for Alteon compound number 711. ('We haven't chosen a real name for it,' Egan told me. 'We're currently playing around with some Latin derivatives – the usual game.')

According to data Alteon have submitted to the US Food and Drug Administration, ALT-711 cuts glycosolation cross-links in animal tests, in one experiment making the coronary ventricles of dogs more supple, in another restoring aged rat skin to youthful elasticity in three days. The drug wasn't toxic in these tests, and it didn't destroy the desirable non-glucose cross-links that help hold collagen together. Some time around the spring of 1998 Egan's group will have submitted an application to the FDA for initial trials of the drug in elderly humans. Egan also envisions a cream-based form of the drug, applied topically to skin.

So look for ALT-711, or whatever sexy Latinate name Alteon decides to give it, at pharmacies and cosmetics counters early in the new milleunium.

*   *   *

---

* The walls of arteries are themselves increasingly cross-linked with age, so a drug that inhibits cross-links may also help to prevent vascular disease by directly softening those arteries, perhaps making them more resistant to the accumulation of cholesterol plaques.

Bodily gunk may be a relatively soluble problem, but the problem of DNA errors – arguably the largest single contributor to ageing – will be much more difficult to overcome. Consider what will be required to keep cellular DNA in a permanently youthful, vigorous state. First, major familial defects that exist at birth will have to be corrected. Second, defects that occur in individual cells in the ordinary course of life (from free radicals, from mutations during cell doubling, etc.) also will have to be corrected.

But where is the technology that will enable us to go into our DNA – cell by cell, for tens of billions of cells, down into every chromosome and mitochondrion – and recognize even tiny errors, and clean each one up? Already we have the beginnings of technologies that will allow us to transplant organs and tissues relatively easily, and to reverse much of the cross-linking and gunking-up that goes on in the body. We can probably even keep cells dividing indefinitely, if we want to, by pumping them with telomerase. But how do we go into cells and effect a detailed manipulation of DNA?

The hard truth is that we can't.

Scientists have been fooling crudely with human DNA *in vivo* – that is, DNA in living cells in the body – for the last ten years, in experiments with 'gene therapy'. The idea of gene therapy has been to remedy genetic diseases or other unwanted conditions by inserting genes into the DNA of cells. The cells then produce the therapeutic proteins for which the new genes code.

Some gene therapy experiments have been promising, and there is little doubt that the technique will play a major role in the medicine of the next couple of decades. But most gene therapy trials so far have been disappointing, a fact which the hype about gene therapy has tended to obscure.

The problem is that scientists have not found a way to get thera-peutic genes into the cells of living people, at least not efficiently. The typical method has been to use a virus, because viruses have been designed by Evolution to carry their own genes into cells and switch those genes on.

Some viruses, such as retroviruses, go so far as to insert their genes into the genomes of the cells they penetrate, thus permanently altering those genomes. But such viruses are tricky. They insert their genes into the genome willy-nilly; there is no telling what gene they will disrupt in the process. That apparently is why retroviruses are associated with cancers: In the process of inscribing themselves into a cell's DNA they destroy tumour-suppressing genes whose job is to keep cell division under control. Without that gene the cell comes a step closer to cancer.

Retroviruses, which include HIV, also have the capability to mutate rapidly. So the practitioners of gene therapy must hobble them, taking out genes here and there to ensure that the virus can't go on a rampage in the body. Unsurprisingly, these neutered viruses aren't very efficient at delivering their genes.

Adenoviruses (a class of DNA viruses that infect respiratory cells and can cause colds) are safer in this respect, and more efficient at infecting cells, but they still have to be hobbled and – more importantly – they don't insert the genes they carry into the chromosomes of cells. They merely set up their own little protein factories within the cytoplasm outside the cell nucleus. And those virus-centred factories can produce proteins only temporarily. So the delivery of genes is only temporary.

In fact, with adenoviruses everything tends to be temporary. Adenoviruses are relatively visible to the immune system, so a cell that produces adenoviral proteins and expresses them on its surface – and this is unavoidable, even when the adenovirus is hobbled – will attract angry T cells that in turn will kill the infected cell, terminating whatever production of therapeutic proteins has been going on within. After repeated doses of adenovirus-delivered gene therapy, which are necessary because each load of genes works only briefly, a patient's immune system will be on constant red alert against the adenoviruses, and will wipe them out before they can deliver their goods.

'Antisense' technology, which has attracted a lot of media coverage in the past few years, seems to offer more precision in DNA targeting, if not more efficiency. In the antisense approach, small strands of nucleotides are injected into the body without any viral packaging; they then find their way into cells and block the activity of the DNA to whose sequence they fit. The idea is to create a variety of useful therapies by shutting off specific harmful genes. It remains to be seen whether this will work – the first generation of antisense drugs failed miserably, and the second are still in early clinical trials – but perhaps one day a similar technology can be used to target specific gene sequences not just for blockage but for repair.

In any case, right now the tools that will enable us to put a desired stretch of genetic material, functionally, into a specific place in the genome of a cell just don't exist. Moreover there are no good techniques for stripping an error-filled stretch of DNA out of a cell's genome, *in vivo*. But if we want to repair every cell in the body, every one of those hundreds of billions of membrane-clad bits of protoplasm, and we want to repair congenital problems as well as the random errors acquired during life, then we must be able to do both: strip out a given stretch of DNA where we want, and then insert new or repaired DNA in the same place. And we must do it 'on the fly', while the cell is still alive and working.

Looking at it this way, I wonder if the repair of DNA, gene by gene, will ever be a solution to the problem of ageing-related DNA errors. It seems much too complicated.

Perhaps a simpler method will be to replace all the DNA in every cell at once. Imagine, for example, giving a DNA sample – a quick swab from your cheek – to a nurse in a clinic. And the cells in that swab are processed to yield up an infinitesimal glob of DNA. And the DNA is sequenced automatically by a machine in the corner, and the computer notifies the clinic what repairs need to be made. And you can specify any other changes you want. And on the basis of all this data another machine synthesizes your new chromosomes. And you lie down and are put to sleep by a doctor and when you wake, a week later, a giant virus-like thing, carrying your new chromosomes, has gone through every cell in your body, organ by organ, removing the old set of chromosomes and inserting the new and improved set.

Or if that is too involved, perhaps scientists can make use of stem cells to replenish your body with youth. Though a bit closer in lineage to ordinary mortal cells, stem cells are like germline cells in that they are multipotential; they have the capacity to bubble off many kinds of differentiated 'daughter' cell. And some seem to have the capacity to do this forever, or at least for a very long time.

Stem cell biology is currently one of the hottest areas of biomedical research. Scientists are trying to perfect techniques to isolate stem cells (which are hard to isolate), and to grow them in culture (they are hard to culture), and already experiments have been performed in which stem-like neural cells – taken controversially from aborted foetuses – have been injected into the brains of human Parkinson's disease patients, to try to replenish dopamine.

Those experiments were crude, and had little success. But some day, perhaps only one or two decades from now, enough will be known about stem cells that they will begin to be used widely in bodily repair and regeneration. If you have a failing organ, for example, a doctor could harvest some stem cells from it – or harvest some from elsewhere and tinker with their DNA, or hit them with the right chemical growth factors, to make them the right kind of stem cell – and could culture a brand-new new organ from those stem cells in some bubbling tank in the lab, or right in your body, next to your old, dying organ.

And here is another scenario: some of your stem cells are harvested, from here and here and there around your body. And their DNA is sequenced and any errors or unwanted sequences are noted and new and clean synthetic chromosomes, made to order, are inserted into the stem cells in laboratory dishes, and these super stem cells, these little cellular fountains of youth, are injected into your body. And as the other, older cells in your body die, the super stem cells and the daughter cells they spawn come to dominate your cellular population. Youth seeps through your body like rising sap.

And all you will need are a few injections per decade to keep everything in your body young – and perhaps the developmental biologists will eventually find ways to replace, *in situ*, your more mechanical, less reparable bits such as bone and cartilage and tooth and claw, and ear parts, and eye parts – or perhaps for these we will be content to rely upon synthetic implants, which will be superior, strong and tough and designed in new and imaginative ways.

And perhaps by the time this all comes to pass some deep thinker somewhere, some ponderer of consciousness, will invent a way to download us all into a new world of computer-driven virtual reality – and we will live for ever, beyond the fleshly killing fields of death, having literally become, at last, the stuff that dreams are made of.

And I am thirty-four. Another year older since I began this book. Will I live for ever? I am afraid to say; I don't want to tempt fate. But I am much more hopeful, at least about staying youthful longer, than I was on that November day when I came through the desert to Sun City. I think differently. I hear politicians worrying about Social Security, and how the baby boomers will all retire in thirty years and swamp the system – and I want to stop them. I want to say: Wait! Ask yourselves – What if, in thirty years, baby boomers are still too youthful and vigorous to retire? What if technology has made everyone youthful who chooses to be, or can afford it? What if our old assumptions about the cycle of life, the passage from cradle to grave, the actuarial tables that relate age to risk of disease and death – what if all these have to be thrown out? What if there is no longer any hard limit to life? What if people, instead of dying, instead choose periodically to overhaul their lives, to change careers, spouses, personalities? What if no one really retires except the lazy?

What if most people *have* to keep working, to be able to pay for all the amazing life-extension products science wants to sell them!

When I set out to write this book I decided to write it not so much for the aged reader as for those from my own generation, at the young end of the baby boom. We have a few decades yet before we start to really worry, seriously worry, about the process of ageing. We have a few decades in which we can sit back and let the scientists devise their amazing cures for death.

Whereas others – parents, relatives, elderly friends – are up against it now. The technologies I have discussed in the last pages will probably not come soon enough for them. Probably the only option now, for an elderly person seeking physical immortality, will be to turn to those flaky Californians I mentioned in the prologue, to have done what only a few dozen people so far have dared to have done. Which is to say they can have their heads cut off after death, and frozen in liquid nitrogen, the hope being that – despite the horrendous damage such freezing causes to brain tissue, with present cryonics technology – their brains might nevertheless be repaired some day, their bodies regenerated, the electric surge of life reinstated, their long sleep ended.

On the other hand, most elderly folk today are not flaky Californians. They do not yearn for physical immortality. Perhaps without wanting to think about it much, they accept death.

I remember shivering, the afternoon I arrived in Sun City, beside a large yellow John Deere backhoe tractor. Temporarily unmanned, it rested before the neat-edged hole it had just finished digging in a quiet corner of Sunland Memorial Cemetery. The sun, looking glum, stared from behind high autumn clouds of ice, its pale heat whipped away jealously by the wind before it could warm anything. The adjacent grave had already been filled, the year before, by Mrs M –, and the grass had healed over. Her birth date and death date were neatly inscribed on the polished face of the large grey gravestone, and her husband, Mr M –, after having delayed a while in the aboveground world of the living, was now about to descend and lie beside her, and there would be a quiet service, or perhaps no service other than the simple lowering of the coffin, guided by ropes and pulleys.

Sunland Memorial sold plots and gravestones in advance and I noted something that future generations might find strange and sad: Mr M –, while still alive, had had his own name inscribed on the stone, his birthday included, an etched line reaching out to touch a clean, blank space – signifying the calm expectancy of his own extinction, the only question being the exact date it would occur.

Acknowledgements

I could not have written this book without the generous cooperation and assistance of 'Max Weller', Joe Rogers, Pat McGeer, Dennis Selkoe, Carl June, Dave Harlan, Allan Kirk,' Peter Linsley, Jeff Ledbetter, Craig Thompson, George Martin, and Jerry Schellenberg. I'm also grateful to Robin Holliday and Steven Austad, whose books *Understanding Ageing* and *Why We Age* moved me quickly up from the bottom of the learning curve.

Source Notes

Phase One: Forever Old

Chapter Three: Inflammation

26   Alzheimer's incidence: Katzman, Aronson, Fuld 1989.
26   Alois Alzheimer: Bick 1994.
29   Lancet article: Davies and Maloney 1976.
30   somatostatin: Morrison, Rogers et al 1985. See also: Davies, Katzman, and Terry 1980.
31   'caused by abnormalities in chemical messengers': Hunt 1991
34   Rogers's thwarted paper: Rogers, Singer et al 1986.

Chapter Four: Voices in the Wilderness

37   Neurobiology of Aging paper: Rogers, Luber-Narod, et al 1988.
38   Cold Spring Harbor: McGeer, Itagaki et al 1988.
40   Four London physicians: Jenkinson, Bliss et al 1988.
41   their own study of hospital data: McGeer, McGeer et al 1990
41–2   Japanese lepers: McGeer, Harada et al 1992.
42   Sun City and Vancouver autopsies: McGeer and McGeer et al 1990.
43   dapsone-soaked brains: Namba, Kawatsu et al 1992.
43   contrary study from Mayo: Beard, Kokman and Kurland 1991.

Chapter Five: The Harvard Baptist

47–8   Selkoe and tau: Yen, Gaskin, and Terry 1981. Selkoe, Ihara, et al, 1982.

48   Finding beta amyloid: Glenner and Wong 1984
50   APP: Kang, Lemaire et al 1987.
51   Selkoe the evangelist: as a science journalist covering Alzheimer's
        I was on the receiving end of some of this in the early '90s.
51   Cotman: Whitson, Selkoe and Cotman 1989.
51   Yankner papers: Yankner, Dawes et al 1989. Yankner, Duffy,
        and Kirschner 1990.
52   Watson and Crick line: Marx 1992
53   mice that overexpressed beta amyloid: Selkoe 1991.
53   lightning struck: Selkoe 1991; Kawabata, Higgins, Gordon
        1991
54   loose ends: Marx 1992b, Schnabel 1993b.
55   rancor: Marx 1992b; this is also my own recollection from
        conversations with Alzheimer's researchers in those days.
55   chromosome 21 defects rare: Alzheimer's genetic findings are
        summarized in Selkoe 1997. general suspicion, retraction of
        mouse paper: Marx 1992a; Kawabata, Higgins, Gordon 1992.

Chapter Six: MAC Attack

62   amyloid and complement paper: Rogers, Cooper et al 1992.
67   prednisone dangers: Wolkowitz, Reus et al 1990.
68   indomethacin trial: Rogers, Kirby et al 1993; Schnabel 1993a,
        1993b.

Chapter Seven: The Finish Line

73   anti–inflammatory hypothesis orthodox now: Breitner, Welsh
        et al 1995; Meda, Cassatella et al 1995.
73   Selkoe's review article: Selkoe 1997.
74   anti–oxidant study: Sano, Ernesto et al 1997.
74   Leber: Drachman and Leber 1997.
74–5   Allen Roses's work: Schmechel, Saunders et al 1993; Strittmatter,
        Saunders et al. 1993.

Chapter Eight: The Wall

83   CholestaGel: Gibbs 1997.
85   angiogenesis inhibitors: Clark 1997; see also the 18 May issue
        of *Time*.

85   Burnham Institute: Barinaga 1997.
86   tk/gancyclovir: Clark 1997.
85–6   gene therapy: Gibbs 1997b; Clark 1997.

Phase Two: Spare Parts

Chapter Ten: The Secret Handshake

110   June's and Ledbetter's work: June, Ledbetter et al 1987.

Chapter Eleven: The Ligand

117   Aruffo and Seed: Aruffo and Seed 1987.
121   Linsley finds that B7 is a ligand for CD28: Linsley, Clark, and
        Ledbetter 1990.

Chapter Twelve: The Blocker

127   Linsley finds that CTLA4 also binds to B7: Linsley, Brady,
        et al 1991.
128   big splash over animal tests: Linsley, Wallace, et al 1992;
        Lenschow, Zeng, et al 1992; Waldholtz 1992; Cohen 1992.

Chapter Thirteen: The Grail

130   Medawar's mice: Billingham, Brent, and Medawar 1953.
132   Naji's mice: Posselt, Barker, et al 1990; Skerett 1990.
134   Jenkins and Schwartz: Jenkins and Schwartz 1987; Jenkins,
        Mueller et al 1991.
136   CTLA4 summary: See for example Chambers, Krummel et
        al 1996.
140   CTLA4Ig monkey failure: Cabrian, Berry, et al 1996.

Chapter Fourteen: Twelve Monkeys

150   Chris Larsen paper: Larsen, Elwood et al 1996.
150   Grewal paper: Grewal, Xu, and Flavell 1995

Chapter Fifteen: We Can All Go Home Now

158   Kirk and Harlan's paper: Kirk, Harlan et al 1997.

Chapter Sixteen: The Selfish Self

163   xenotransplantation: Butler 1998; Rhodes 1997.
165   Xenopus: Holiday 1995.
166   regeneration: see the special issue of *Science*, 4 April 1997.

Phase Three: Forever Young

Chapter Seventeen: The Gray Gene

171   Helen: Epstein, Martin, Schultz, and Motulsky 1966.

Chapter Eighteen: The Race

177–8 muscular dystrophy story: Wingerson 1990.
181   Goto/Drayna's first paper: Goto, Rubinstein et al 1992.

Chapter Nineteen: The Markers

183   Lancet paper: Schellenberg, Martin et al 1992.
187   Winston Thomas paper: Thomas, Rubinstein, Goto, and
       Drayna 1993.
189   1994 papers: Yu, Oshima et al 1994.

Chapter Twenty: The Gene Cleaner

195   Werner's gene paper: Yu, Oshima et al 1996.
197–   Hayflick limits, telomeres: Holliday 1995; Austad 1997; Hawley
200   1997; Barinaga 1997; Brown, Wei, and Sedivy 1997; Bodnar,
       Ouelette et al 1998; De Lange 1998.
202   glycosolation, AGEs: Holliday 1995; Vasan, Zhang, et al 1996.
204   gene therapy: a nice review is found in Clark 1997.
205   antisense: Clark 1997; Roush 1997.
206   stem cells: special issue of *Science*, 4 April 1997; Clark 1997.

Bibliography

Aruffo, A, and Seed, B.

1987. Molecular cloning of a CD28 cDNA by a high efficiency COS cell expression system. *Proceedings of the National Academy of Sciences* 84: 8573–77.

Austad, Steven

1997. Why we age. New York: Wiley.

Barinaga, M.

1997. The telomerase picture fills in. *Science* 276: 528–9.

1998. Peptide-guided cancer drugs show promise in mice. *Science* 279: 323–4.

Beard, C.M., Kokman, E., and Kurland, L.

1991. Rheumatoid arthritis and susceptibility to Alzheimer's disease. *Lancet* 337: 1426.

Bick, Katherine L.

1994. The early story of Alzheimer disease. In R.D. Terry, R. Katzman, and K.L. Bick, *Alzheimer Disease*. New York: Raven.

Billingham, R., Brent, L., and Medawar, P.

1953. 'Actively acquired tolerance' of foreign cells. *Nature* 172: 603–6.

Bodnar, A., Ouellette, M., *et al.*

1998. Extension of life-span by introduction of telomerase into normal human cells. *Science* 279: 349–52.

Breitner, J., Welsh, K., *et al.*

1995. Delayed onset of Alzheimer's disease with nonsteroidal anti-inflammatory and histamine H2 blocking drugs. *Neurobiology of Ageing* 16: 523–30.

Bretscher, P., and Cohn, M.

1970. [to follow]. *Science* [to follow]: [to follow]

Brown, J., Wei, W., and Sedivy, J.

1997. Bypass of senescence after disruption of p21CIP1/WAF1 gene in normal diploid human fibroblasts. *Science* 277: 831–3.

Butler, D.

1998. Briefing: xenotransplantation. *Nature* 391: 320–5.

Cabrian, K., Berry, K., *et al.*

1996. Suppression of T-cell dependent immune responses in monkeys by CTLA4Ig. *Transplantation Proceedings*. 28: 3261–2

Chambers, C., Krummel, M., et al.

1996. The role of CTLA-4 in the regulation and initiation of T-cell responses. *Immunological Reviews* 153: 27–46.

Clark, W.

1997. *The new healers*. New York: Oxford University Press.

Cohen, J.

1992. Mounting a targeted strike on unwanted immune responses. *Science* 257: 751.

Davies, P., and Maloney, A.

1976. Selective loss of central cholinergic neurons in Alzheimer's disease. *Lancet* ii, 1403.

Davies, P., Katzman, R., and Terry, R.

1980. Reduced somatostatin-like immunoreactivity in cerebral cortex from cases of Alzheimer disease and Alzheimer senile dementia. *Nature* 288: 279–80.

De Lange, T.

1998. Telomeres and senescence: ending the debate. *Science* 279: 334–5.

Drachman, D., and Leber, P.

1997. Treatment of Alzheimer's disease – searching for a breathrough, settling for less. *New England Journal of Medicine* 336: 1245–7.

Epstein, C., Martin, G., Schultz, A., and Motulsky, A.

1966. Werner's syndrome. *Medicine* 45: 177–221.

Gibbs, W.

1997a. Dredging the digestive system. *Scientific American* (April): 38.
1997b. A cold for cancer. *Scientific American* (August): 23–4.

Glenner, G., and Wong, C.

1984. Alzheimer's disease: initial report of the purification and characterization of a novel cerebrovascular amyloid protein. *Biochemical and Biophysiological Research Communications* 120: 885–90

Goto, M., Rubenstein, M., et al.

1992. Genetic linkage of Werner's syndrome to five markers on chromosome 8. *Nature* 355: 735–8.

Goto, M., Tanimoto, K. et al.

1981. Family analysis of Werner's syndrome: a survey of 42 Japanese families with a review of the literature. *Clinical Genetics* 19: 8–15.

Grewal, I., Xu, J., and Flavell, R.

1995. Impairment of antigen-specific T-cell priming in mice lacking CD40 ligand. *Nature* 378: 617–20.

Gura, T.

1997. How TRAIL kills cancer cells, but not normal cells. *Science* 277: 768.

Hawley, R.

1997. Sticky endings: separating telomeres. *Science* 276: 1215.

Holliday, Robin

1995. *Understanding ageing*. New York: Cambridge University Press.

Hunt, Liz

1991. Drug offers hope for Alzheimer's sufferers. *Independent*, 26 April.

Jenkins, M., Mueller, D., *et al.*

1991. Induction and maintenance of anergy in mature T cells. In *Mechanisms of Lymphocyte Activation and Immune Regulation* III, ed. S. Gupta *et al.* New York: Plenum Press. pp. 167–76.

Jenkins, M., and Schwartz, R.

1987. Antigen presentation by chemically modified splenocytes induces antigen-specific T cell unresponsiveness *in vitro* and *in vivo*. *Journal of Experimental Medicine* 165: 302–19.

Jenkinson, M., Bliss, M., et al.

1988. Rheumatoid arthritis and senile dementia of the Alzheimer's type. *British Journal of Rheumatology* 28: 86–7.

June, C., Ledbetter, J., *et al.*

1987. T-cell proliferation involving the CD28 pathway is associated with cyclosporine-resistant Interleukin-2 gene expression. *Molecular and Cellular Biology* 7: 4472–81.

Kang, J., Lemaire, H.G., *et al.*

1987. The precursor of Alzheimer's disease amyloid-A4 protein resembles a cell surface receptor. *Nature* 325: 733–6.

Katzman, R., Aronson, M., Fuld, P, et al.,

1989. Development of dementing illnesses in an 80-year old volunteer cohort. *Annals of Neurology* 25: 317–24

Kawabata, S., Higgins, G., and Gordon, J.

1991. Amyloid plaques, neurofibrillary tangles and neuronal loss in brains of transgenic mice overexpressing a C-terminal fragment of human amyloid precursor protein. *Nature* 354: 476–78.

1992. Alzheimer's retraction. *Nature* 356: 23.

Kirk, A., Harlan, D., *et al.*

1997. CTLA4-Ig and anti-CD40 ligand prevent renal allograft rejection in primates. *Proceedings of the National Academy of Sciences* 94: 8789–94.

Larsen, C., Elwood, E., et al.

1996. Long-term acceptance of skin and cardiac allografts after blocking CD40 and CD28 pathways. *Nature* 381: 434–8.

Lanzavecchia, A.

1998. License to kill. *Nature* 393: 413–14

Lenschow, D., Zeng, Y., *et al.*

1992. Long-term survival of xenogeneic pancreatic islet grafts induced by CTLA4Ig. *Science* 257: 789–92.

Linsley, P., Brady, W., *et al.*

1991. CTLA-4 is a second receptor for the B cell activation antigen B7. *Journal of Experimental Medicine* 174: 561–7.

Linsley, P., Clark, E., and Ledbetter, J.

1990. T-cell antigen CD28 mediates adhesion with B cells by interacting with activation antigen B7/BB-1. *Proceedings of the National Academy of Sciences* 87: 5031–5.

Linsley, P., Wallace, P., *et al.*

1992. Immunosuppression in vivo by a soluble form of the CTLA-4 T cell activation molecule. *Science* 257: 792–5.

Luber-Narod, J., and Rogers, J.

1988. Immune system associated antigens expressed by cells of the human central nervous system. *Neuroscience Letters* 94: 17–22.

McGeer, P., Harada, N., *et al.*

1992. Prevalence of dementia amongst elderly Japanese with leprosy: apparent effect of chronic drug therapy. *Dementia* 3: 146–9.

McGeer, P., Itagaki, S., *et al.*

1988. Immune system response in Alzheimer's disease. In C. Finch and P. Davies, *The Molecular Biology of Alzheimer's Disease*. Cold Spring Harbor Laboratory.

McGeer, P., McGeer, E., Rogers, J., and Sibley, J.

1990. Anti-inflammatory drugs and Alzheimer's disease. *Lancet* 335: 1037.

Marx, J.

1992a. Major setback for Alzheimer's models. *Science* 255: 1200–1201.
1992b. Alzheimer's debate boils over. *Science* 257: 1336–8.

Meda, L., Cassatella, M., *et al.*

1995. Activation of microglial cells by beta amyloid and interferon gamma. *Nature* 374: 647–50.

Morrison, J., Rogers, J., *et al.*

1985. Somatostatin immunoreactivity in neuritic plaques of Alzheimer's patients. *Nature*: 314: 90–92.

Nakura, J., Wijsman, E., *et al.*

1994. Homozygosity mapping of the Werner syndrome locus. *Genomics* 23: 600–608.

Namba, Y., Kawatsu, K., *et al.*

1992. Neurofibrillary tangles and senile plaques in brains of elderly leprosy patients. *Lancet* 340: 978–9.

Oshima, J., Yu, C., *et al.*

1994. Integrated mapping analysis of the Werner syndrome region of chromosome 8. *Genomics* 23: 100–113.

Posselt, A., Barker, C., *et al.*

1990. Induction of donor-specific unresponsiveness by intrathymic islet transplant. *Science* 249: 1293–5.

Rhodes, R.

1997. *Deadly Feasts*. New York: Simon and Schuster.

Rogers, J., Cooper, N., Webster, S., *et al.*

1992. Complement activation by beta-amyloid in Alzheimer disease. *Proceedings of the National Academy of Sciences* 89: 10016–20.

Rogers, J., Kirby, L., *et al.*

1993. Clinical trial of indomethacin in Alzheimer's disease. *Neurology* 43: 1609–11.

Rogers, J., Luber-Narod, J., et al.

1988. Expression of immune system associated antigens by cells of the human central nervous system: relationship to the pathology of Alzheimer's disease. *Neurobiology of Aging* 9: 339–49.

Rogers, J., Singer, R.H., *et al.*

1986. Neurovirologic and neuroimmunologic considerations in Alzheimer's disease. *Society for Neuroscience Abstracts* 12: 944.

Roush, W.

1997. Antisense aims for a renaissance. *Science* 276: 1192–3.

Sano, M., Ernesto, C., et al.

1997. A controlled trial of selegeline, alpha-tocopherol, or both as treatment for Alzheimer's disease. *New England Journal of Medicine* 336: 1216–47.

Schellenberg, G.D., et al.

1992. Genetic linkage evidence for a familial Alzheimer's disease locus on chromosome 14. *Science* 258: 668–71.

Schellenberg, G., Martin, G., *et al.*

1992. Homozygosity mapping and Werner's syndrome. *Lancet* 339: 1002.

Schmechel, D., Saunders, A., *et al.*

1993. Increased amyloid beta-peptide deposition in cerebral cortex as a consequence of apolipoprotein E genotype in late-onset Alzheimer disease. *Proceedings of the National Academy of Sciences* 90: 9649–53.

Schnabel, J.

1993a. New Alzheimer's therapy suggested. *Science* 260: 1719–20.

1993b. Alzheimer's disease: arthritis of the brain? *New Scientist*, 19 June, 22–6.

Selkoe, D.

1991. In the beginning. *Nature* 354: 432–3.

1997. Alzheimer's disease: genotypes, phenoype, and treatments. *Science* 275: 630–31.

Selkoe, D., Abraham, C., *et al.*

1984. Isolation of low molecular weight proteins from amyloid plaque fibers in Alzheimer's disease. *Journal of Neurochemistry*. 146: 1820–34.

Selkoe, D., Ihara, Y., *et al.*

1982. Alzheimer's disease: insolubility of partially purified paired helical filaments in sodium dodecyl sulfate and urea. *Science* 215: 1243–5.

Selkoe, D., Abraham, C., *et al.*

1985. Isolation of low molecular weight proteins from amyloid plaque fibers in Alzheimer's disease. *Journal of Neurochemistry* 46: 1820–34.

Skerett, P.

1990. New transplant method evades immune attack. *Science* 249: 1248.

Stipp, D.

1990. Alzheimer's study suggests brain chemical is culprit. *Wall Street Journal*, 12 October.

St George-Hyslop, P., *et al.*

1987. *Science* 235: 885.

1992. *Nature Genetics* 2: 330–34.

Strittmatter, W., Saunders, A., *et al.*

1993. Apolipoprotein-E: high avidity binding to beta amyloid and increased frequency of type 4 allele in late-onset familial Alzheimer's disease. *Proceedings of the National Academy of Sciences* 90: 1977–81.

Thannhauser, S.

1945. Werner's syndrome (progeria of the adult) and Rothmund's syndrome. *Annals of Internal Medicine* 23: 559–626.

Thomas, W., Rubenstein, M., Goto, M., and Drayna, D.

1993. A genetic analysis of the Werner syndrome region on human chromosome 8p. *Genomics* 16: 685–90.

Van Essen, D., Kikutani, H., and Gray, D.

1995. CD40 ligand-transduced co-stimulation of T-cells in the development of helper function. *Nature* 378: 620–23.

Vasan, S., Zhang, X., *et al.*

1996. An agent cleaving glucose-derived protein crosslinks in vitro and in vivo. *Nature* 382: 275–8.

Waldholtz, M.

1992. Bristol-Myers drug holds hope for organ transplants. *Wall Street Journal*, 7 August.

Whitson, J., Selkoe, D., and Cotman, C.

1989. Amyloid beta protein enhances the survival of hippocampal neurons in vitro. *Science* 243: 1488–90.

Wingerson, Lois.

1990. *Mapping our genes*. New York: Plume.

Wolkowitz, O., Reus, V., *et al.*

1990. Cognitive effects of corticosteroids. *American Journal of Psychiatry* 147: 1297–1303.

Yankner, B., Dawes, L., *et al.*

1989. Neurotoxicity of a fragment of the amyloid precursor associated with Alzheimer's disease. *Science* 245: 417–20.

Yankner, B., Duffy, L., and Kirschner, D.

1990. Neurotrophic and neurotoxic effects of amyloid beta protein: reversal by tachykinin neuropeptides. *Science* 250: 279–82.

Yen, S., Gaskin, F., and Terry R.

1981. Immunocytochemical studies of neurofibrillary tangles. *American Journal of Pathology* 104: 77–89.

Yu, C., Oshima, J. *et al.*

1994. Linkage disequilibrium and haplotype studies of chromosome 8p 11.1–21.1 markers and Werner syndrome. *American Journal of Human Genetics* 55: 356–64.

Yu, C., Oshima, J. *et al.*

1996. Positional cloning of the Werner's syndrome gene. *Science* 272: 258–62.

Index

Abraham, Carmela, 48
Agene, 188
ageing, current theories of, 87–89
Alteon Inc., 202–3
Alzheimer, Alois, 26–7
Alzheimer's disease:
  acetylcholine hypothesis
    and, 28–31
  aluminium hypothesis and, 32
  amyloid hypothesis and, 32, 44–60
  Apo-E4 and, 74–6
  antioxidants and, 74
  complement activation in, 61–5
  diagnosis of, 10–13
  oestrogen levels and risk of, 76
  early-onset form of, 26–7,
    50–1, 55–6
  inflammation hypothesis and,
    40–4, 60, 73
  mouse models of, 53–4, 56–9
  neurofibrillary tangles in, 26,
    31–2, 46–8
  prevalence of, 25–6
  viruses and, 32–39
Aricept, 74
Aruffo, Alejandro, 117
Athena Neuroscience, 45, 55, 76, 79
atherosclerosis (see vascular disease)

B7, 123–43

Beatty, Patrick, 109–10
Beyreuther, Konrad, 49
Billingham, Rupert, 130
Biogen, 152, 159
Blackburn, Elizabeth, 198
Bluestone, Jeffrey, 127, 138, 149
bone marrow transplants, 95–106
Bovine spongiform encephalopathy
  (BSE), 19n
Brachova, Libuse, 15–21
Brady, Bill, 124
Brent, Leslie, 130
Bretscher, Peter, 134n
Bristol Myers Squibb, 137–41
Bryer, Bruce, 177–78

Cancer:
  angiogenesis inhibitors and, 84–5
  gene therapy and, 85–6
CD4Ig, 124, 125n
CD28 (Tp44), 113–135
CD40, 150–9
CholestaGel, 83
chronic granulomatous disease, 178
chronic myelocytic leukemia, 95
cloning, 163
Cognex, 74
Cohn, Mel 134n
Cold Spring Harbor Laboratories, 38
Cooper, Neil, 62–4

Cotman, Carl, 51–2
Creutzfeldt-Jacob disease, 19, 164
CRM-19, 146–47
CTLA4 (CD152), 125–50
Culver, Kenneth, 86
cyclosporine, 101–110

dapsone, 41–2
Darwin, Charles, 169
Darwin Molecular, 191
DNA:
    accumulation of errors in,
        194–201
    keeping clean, 204–6
dopamine, 28–9
Down's Syndrome, 50
Drachman, David, 29–30
Drayna, Dennis, 179–88

Eccles, Sir John, 40
Egan, Jack, 203
Eikelenboom, Piet, 44
Einstein, Albert, 169
Eli Lilly & Co., 76, 79
Epstein, Charles, 172, 174

Finch, Caleb 'Tuck', 38, 44
5C8, 152–164
free radicals, 74
freezing brains, 3, 208

gancyclovir, 86
graft-versus-host disease, 100–4
GelTex Pharmaceuticals, 83
Genentech Corp., 123–4, 125n
gene therapy, 85–6, 204–5
Genetics Institute, 138, 146, 152
Geron Corp, 199
glycosolation, 201–3
Golstein, Pierre, 125
'Good Morning America', 158
Gordon, Jon, 57, 59

Goto, Makato, 179–88, 192
Grewal, Iqbal, 150
Greider, Carol, 198
Gusella, Jim, 50

Hansen, John, 109–12
Harlan, Dave, 142–4, 149–52,
    155, 157–9
Harlem Globetrotters, 39
Harley, Calvin, 199
Hayflick, Leonard, 175
Hayflick limit, 175–6, 197–8
helicases, 194–95
Higgins, Gerald, 56–9
Hiteshew, Doug, 94
Howard Hughes Institute, 125, 138
Hutchinson Cancer Research
    Center 95–113

Ihara, Yasuo, 47
indomethacin, 68–71
'Ishiguro' family, 171–73

Jenkins, Marc, 134–35, 139
June, Carl,
    background, 93–4
    at Hutchinson Center, 95–118,
        125
    at Navy lab in Bethesda, 143,
        149, 155

Kawabata, Shigeki, 53, 59
Khachaturian, Zaven, 60
Kinsella, Kevin, 45, 49
Kirk, Allan, 144–59
Knechtle, Stuart, 144–5, 153
Kohler, Georges, 111
Kolata, Gina, 49
Kunkel, Louis, 177–8
kuru, 19n

Larsen, Chris, 150–1

Leber, Paul, 74
Ledbetter, Jeffrey, 110–13, 116–27, 134, 141
Lee, Virginia, 76
Lenschow, Debbie, 128–9, 137–9
Lieberburg, Ivan, 64, 70
life expectancy, human, 83, 86
Lindsten, Tullia, 125
Linsley, Peter, 116–29, 135, 137–41
Lue, Lih-Fen, 16–21

McGeer, Edith, 40
McGeer, Patrick, 37–44, 61, 64–5, 68, 72–3, 80
Martin, George, 172–83
Martin, Paul, 109–10
Marx, Jean, 49
Massachusetts General Hospital, 117
Mayo Clinic, 43
Medawar, Peter, 130–1, 155
Mercator Genetics, 188
Miki, Tetsuro, 186
Milstein, Cesar, 111
misoprostol, 73
monoclonal antibodies, 111
'Morderas, Maria', 95–104
'Morton, Edgar', 14–21
Motulsky, Arno, 172
muscular dystrophy, 177–8

Naji, Ali, 132–33
nerves, regeneration of, 165
Non-steroidal anti-inflammatory drugs (NSAIDs), 68–73

Oncogen, 116, 137–38
organ donations, 162–63

Parkinson's disease, 28–9
Perl, Dan, 32
Pfizer, 74
Picower Institute, 202–03

polymerase chain reaction, 184n
prednisone, 66–8, 72, 105

repeat markers, 183–90
Repligen Corp., 138
restriction enzymes, 176–77
retinitis pigmentosa, 178
Rogers, Joe,
    early years, 23–5
    grad school 25
    at U-Mass 29–35
    in Sun City 13–23, 35–7
    starts collaboration with McGeer 38–44, 60–73, 80–1

St George-Hyslop, Peter, 50
Salk Institute, 25
Sandoz, 101, 105
Schellenberg, Gerard, 178–95
Schwartz, Ron, 134–35
secretase (alpha, beta, gamma), APP, 50, 78–9
Seed, Brian, 117
Selkoe, Dennis, 32, 45–59, 73, 77–80
Shapiro, Ron, 158
Slack, Jonathan, 164
Society for Neuroscience 35, 37
Sollinger, Hans, 144, 146
spare parts, concept of in future medicine, 113–16
stem cells, 206–7
Sue, Lucia, 15–21
'Sullivan, Herbert,' 66–7
Sun City, 3–6, 9–22, 35–6, 41, 65–71, 73, 81, 207–9

Tanzi, Rudi, 50
TCR (T-cell receptor), 101
telomeres, 197–201
Terry, Bob, 47–48
Thannhauser, S.J. 174
Thomas, E. Donnal 'Don', 109–10

Thomas, Winston, 186–87
Thompson, Craig, 125, 138
thymidine kinase, 86
tolerance (immunological):
   fetal injection experiment, 130–31
   thymic injection experiments,
     132–33
   two-signal theoretical model,
     134–35
   and CTLA4Ig, 135–36
   and CD40 blockers, 159
transplant, organ:
   common in future, 162
   current frequency in USA, 162
   monkey experiments, 143–56
   need for immunosuppression, 102
   organs grown in labs, 163
   waiting list for, 162
   xenotransplants, 163–65
Trojanowski, John, 76–7

Ulrich, Peter, 203
Upjohn, 83

vascular disease, 83–4
Warner-Lambert, 74
Webster, Scott 16–21, 63
'Weller, Max' 9–13, 70–1
'Weller, Mildred' 9–13, 70–1
Weiner, Howard, 49
Werner, Otto, 174
Werner's syndrome:
   discovery, 174
   features, 171–76
   helicase function of gene mutated
     in, 194–95
   prevalence, 172, 179–180
   race to find gene for, 178–94
Whitson, Janet, 51–2
Wisniewski, Henry, 59

Xenopus, 165

Yankner, Bruce, 51–5
Yu, Chang-En, 188–93